W9-BEN-285

Family in America

Family in America

Advisory Editors: David J. Rothman

**Professor of History,
Columbia University**

Sheila M. Rothman

PSYCHOLOGICAL CARE

OF

INFANT AND CHILD

By

JOHN B. WATSON, Ph. D.

With the Assistance of
ROSALIE RAYNER WATSON

ᴀRNO ᴘRESS & ᴛHE ɴEW ʏORK ᴛIMES

New York   1972

PSYCHOLOGICAL CARE

OF

INFANT AND CHILD

By

JOHN B. WATSON, Ph. D.

Formerly Professor of Psychology
The Johns Hopkins University
Author of "Behaviorism"

With the Assistance of
ROSALIE RAYNER WATSON

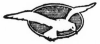

NEW YORK

W·W·NORTON & COMPANY, INC.

Publishers

PRINTED IN THE UNITED STATES OF AMERICA
FOR THE PUBLISHERS BY THE VAIL-BALLOU PRESS

DEDICATED TO THE
FIRST MOTHER WHO
BRINGS UP A HAPPY
CHILD.

CONTENTS

ACKNOWLEDGMENTS

The scientific material, upon which the convictions set forth in this small hand book are based, has been gathered in the Maternity Ward of the Johns Hopkins Hospital, the Harriet Lane Home for Crippled Children, at the Heckscher Foundation, and in many private homes.

In our experimental work at the Johns Hopkins Hospital we received the whole hearted cooperation of Dr. J. Whitridge Williams, Dr. Adolf Meyer, Dr. Kenneth Blackfan, and the late Dr. John Howland.

We are under deep obligations to the Trustees of the Laura Spelman Rockefeller Memorial who by a grant to the Institute of Educational Research of Teacher's College made possible the work of Dr. Mary Cover Jones at the Heckscher Foundation.

2   ACKNOWLEDGMENTS

Many individuals have helped to shape either our work or our conclusions. We are under deepest obligations to Dr. Leslie B. Hohman of Phipps Psychiatric Clinic, The Johns Hopkins Hospital; to Dr. Mary Cover Jones of the Psychology Department of the University of California; Dr. Karl S. Lashley of the Institute for Juvenile Research, Chicago; Dr. Kenneth Blackfan now of the Children's Hospital, Harvard Medical School; Dr. John J. Morgan of Northwestern University; Dr. Alvin Johnson, and Dr. Horace Kallen of the New School for Social Research; Dr. H. M. Johnson of the Mellon Institute; Professor Patty S. Hill, Teachers College; to Dr. George Dorsey and to Dr. W. I. Thomas.

We have received many valuable suggestions on the editorial side from Miss Anne B. Juenker and Miss Janet Cunningham of the J. Walter Thompson Company, and from the editors of McCall's Magazine who published a part of this material.

INTRODUCTION

Ever since my first glimpse of Dr. Holt's "The Care and Feeding of Children," I hoped some day to be able to write a book on the psychological care of the infant. I believed then that psychological care was just as necessary as physiological care. Today I believe it is in some ways more important. Healthy babies do grow up under the most varied form of feeding and bodily care. They can be stunted by poor food and ill health and then in a few days of proper régime be made to pick up their weight and bodily strength.

But once a child's character has been spoiled by bad handling which can be done in a few days, who can say that the damage is ever repaired?

I know this book is not as complete on the psychological side as Dr. Holt's is on the care of the body but the behaviorist does not know enough today to do a thoroly satisfactory job. We have only just begun to believe that there is such a thing as the psychological care of infants and children.

A great many mothers still resent being told how to feed their children. Didn't their grandmothers have fourteen children and raise ten of them? Didn't their own mothers have six and eight children and raise them all—and they never needed a doctor to tell them how to feed them? That many of grandmother's children grew up with rickets, with poor teeth, with under-nourished bodies, generally prone to every kind of disease means little to the mother who doesn't want to be told how to feed her child scientifically. But thousands of mothers have found in Dr. Holt something as valuable as the Bible. The 28 editions of his work abundantly prove this.

Parents—mothers especially—resent still more strenuously any advice or instructions on how to care psychologically for their children. What parents want advice on how much affection they should bestow upon their children or any word about how their children should be handled and treated hourly in the home? "I can't take my child up in my lap! I can't let my children sleep together! I can't let my child play around me all I want to! I can't slap him or scold him if I care to! I have to begin talking sex to him the moment he is born! Who ever heard of such a thing?" And do not think this is a backwoods attitude. On the main streets of every city, village and town you find just such parents. You find the same resistance in the homes of college professors and in the homes even of pediatricians. Even in the homes of "advanced" mothers— mothers who are listening eagerly for words of wisdom about the care of their children you find the complaint— "The behaviorists are on the right track but they go too far."

It is a serious question in my mind whether there should be individual homes for children—or even whether children should know their own parents. There are undoubtedly much more scientific ways of bringing up children which will probably mean finer and happier children. I suppose parents want their children to be happy, efficient, well adjusted to life. But if I were to offer to take any mother's child and guarantee it such an up-bringing, and were even to convince the mother at the same time that she was unques-tionably unfitted to bring up her child—that she would inevitably bring up a weakling, a petted, spoiled, sullen, shy youngster who would grow up a liar and a thief—would she give up the child to me? No, the social pres-sure to have a child, to own a child, to be known in the community as a woman with a legitimate child, is strong—it is a part of our *mores*.

The home we have with us—inevitably and inexorably with us. Even though it is proven unsuccessful, we shall always have it. The behaviorist has to accept the home and make the best of it. His task is to try to get the mother to take a new view of what constitutes the care of an infant—of her responsibility for her experiment in child bearing.

Since the behaviorists find little that corresponds to instincts in children, since children are made not born, failure to bring up a happy child, a well adjusted child—assuming bodily health—falls upon the parents' shoulders. The acceptance of this view makes child-rearing the most important of all social obligations.

Since the most serious faults in the rearing of children are to be found on the emotional side I have put especial emphasis upon the growth of emotional habits. The other two phases taken up are day and night time care and the kind and amount of sex instruction that should be given.

One of the many criticisms which may be argued against the book is the fact that I have written principally to mothers who have leisure to devote to the study of their children. The reason I have chosen these more fortunate mothers as my audience, grows out

of the hope I have that some day the importance of the first two years of infancy will be
fully realized. When it is faced, every woman
will seriously question whether she is in a
proper situation to have a child. Today we
debate whether we can buy a motor car—
whether the house or apartment is big enough
to keep a dog—whether we can afford to belong to a club. But the young mother rarely
questions whether her home can house a child
or whether her husband's salary or weekly
wage will stretch far enough to feed another
incessantly hungry body. No, she has the child
and we all rush to congratulate the pair and
smile and smirk over an occurrence which
takes place two and a half million times each
year in the United States of America. The
having of a child should be a carefully
thought out operation. No mother has a right
to have a child who cannot give it a room to
itself for the first two years of infancy. I
would make this a *conditio sine qua non.*

When the 25 million American homes come

to realize that the child has a right to a separate room and adequate psychological care there will not be nearly so many children born. *Not more babies but better brought up babies* will be our slogan. The idea that our population must sustain itself and show an increase is an old fetish growing out of tribal warfare. Why should we care if the U. S. birth rate begins to decline—even more rapidly than that of France? There are too many people in the world now—too many people with crippled personalities—tied up with such a load of infantile carry-overs (due to faulty bringing up) that they have no chance for happy lives.

The purpose of this small volume will be accomplished abundantly if it contributes in any way to help the serious mother solve the problem of bringing up a happy child—a child who never cries unless actually stuck by a pin, illustratively speaking—who loses himself in work and play—who quickly learns to overcome the small difficulties in his environment without running to mother, father, nurse or other adult—who soon builds up a wealth of habits that tides him over dark and rainy days—who puts on such habits of politeness and neatness and cleanliness that adults are willing to be around him at least part of the day; a child who is willing to be around adults without fighting incessantly for notice —who eats what is set before him and "asks no questions for conscience sake"—who sleeps and rests when put to bed for sleep and rest —who puts away 2 year old habits when the third year has to be faced—who passes into adolescence so well equipped that adolescence is just a stretch of fertile years—and who finally enters manhood so bulwarked with stable work and emotional habits that no adversity can quite overwhelm him.

JOHN B. WATSON

New York
March 1st, 1928

CHAPTER ONE

HOW THE BEHAVIORIST STUDIES INFANTS AND CHILDREN

THE oldest profession of the race today is facing failure. This profession is parenthood. Many thousands of mothers do not even know that parenthood should be numbered among the professions. They do not realize that there are any especial problems involved in rearing children. For them the age-old belief that all that children need is food as often as they call for it, warm clothes and a roof over their heads at night, is enough. "Nature" does the rest almost unaided. They argue that parents have been rearing children for a great many centuries, therefore why bother about learning anything new?

A still larger number of mothers become overly devoted to their children. The earth revolves around them. They give them every

11

care, shower physical comforts upon them.
The children are not allowed to draw a breath
unscrutinized. These mothers are prodigal of
their affection, raining love and tears upon
them constantly. For them love is the keynote
of the psychology of child-rearing.

In happy contrast to these two types of
mothers, there is a third group—the modern
mother who is beginning to find that the rearing of children is the most difficult of all professions, more difficult than engineering, than
law, or even than medicine itself. But along
with this conviction comes the search for facts
which will help them. The search reveals almost a bankruptcy of facts. *No one today
knows enough to raise a child.* The world
would be considerably better off if we were
to stop having children for twenty years (except those reared for experimental purposes)
and were then to start again with enough facts
to do the job with some degree of skill and
accuracy. Parenthood, instead of being an
instinctive art, is a science, the details of

which must be worked out by patient laboratory methods.

Will you believe the almost astounding truth that *no well trained man or woman has ever watched the complete and daily development of a single child from its birth to its third year? Plants and animals we know about because we have studied them, but the human child until very recently has been a mystery*. Radium has had more scientific study put upon it in the last fifteen years than has been given to the first three years of infancy since the beginning of time. How can we get facts on how to rear children unless we make the studies necessary to obtain them?

It is true that mothers since Eve have watched their children come into the world and begin to grow up. They know the child can cry at birth. They know that as time goes on more and more things around the house make it cry. When it cries a hundred times a day, as many millions of them do, we say it is "spoiled." And we put the blame on the child rather than upon our own shoulders where the blame belongs.

The mother knows the infant can smile and gurgle and chuckle with glee. She knows it can coo and hold out its chubby arms. What more touching and sweet, what more thrilling to a young mother! And the mother to get these thrills goes to extreme lengths. She picks the infant up, kisses and hugs it, rocks it, pets it and calls it "mother's little lamb," until the child is unhappy and miserable whenever away from actual physical contact with the mother. Then again as we face this intolerable situation of our own creating, we say the child is "spoiled." And spoiled most children are. Rarely does one see a normal child —a child that is comfortable—a child that adults can be comfortable around—a child more than nine months of age that is constantly happy.

Most mothers perhaps feel quite naturally that all infant and childish activities, whether "good" or "bad," are due to the unfolding of the inborn equipment of the child; and that they as parents haven't much to do with the process of growth.

But in the last few years there has come a social Renaissance, a preparation for a change in *mores*, a scrutiny of age-old customs that bids fair to become much more of an epoch in history than the scientific Renaissance which began with Bacon in the 15th century. This awakening is beginning to show itself in mothers who ask themselves the question, "Am I not almost wholly responsible for the way my child grows up? *Isn't it just possible that almost nothing is given in heredity and that practically the whole course of development of the child is due to the way I raise it?*" When she first faces this thought, she shies away from it as being too horrible. She would rather load this burden upon heredity, upon the Divine shoulder, or upon any shoulder other than her own. Once she faces it, accepts it and begins to stagger under the load, she asks herself the question, "What shall I do? If I am responsible for what this tiny being is to become, where shall I find the light to guide my footsteps?" When such thoughts drive is it any wonder that there has been recently an almost frantic interest in what the laboratories of the behaviorist psychologists have to say about *infant culture?*

Even they can help us all too little. Prejudice against laboratory work upon infants and children has been very strong. Scientific study has been slow in getting under way. But in spite of all prejudice a definite beginning has been made. Work has begun. It promises to yield practical results, results which can be used in the home.

What kind of work? What can we do with newborn infants and young children in a psychological laboratory? What practical conclusions can be drawn from work already done?

The setting for experimental work

To get a picture of what we are doing I shall ask you first to think of a lying-in hospital where 40–50 children are born per month. Near by the ward where the babies are kept there is a psychological laboratory. After the infants are washed and dressed, they are brought to the laboratory and put under observation. They must sleep a great deal so the periods of observation at first are very short. These infants are kept under daily and sometimes hourly observation from birth. Selected infants (those whose mothers are to be kept in the hospital as wet nurses) are retained for observation sometimes for more than a year. In our experiments at the Johns Hopkins Hospital, which mark the beginning of such work, we observed more than five hundred infants. Never once was there a mishap. Infants are really very hardy—not at all the hot house plants they are supposed to be. The

mere physical act of being born and the daily
acts of bathing and dressing them, subject
them to far greater hardships than any they
will later meet in the laboratory.

To make our work more nearly complete
we went into orphanages and made daily or
weekly observations on children from one to
six years of age. Finally, in order to compare
laboratory raised products with the home
raised, we selected a group of children for
study from better class homes.

Possibly the easiest way to give an impres-
sion of the kind of work the behaviorist is
doing is to show actual photographs of some
of the infants undergoing tests. These photographs are enlargements made from the mo-
tion picture study of the work at Hopkins. It
is difficult to make cuts from such enlargements, hence, considerable retouching of the
plates was necessary. No situation or reaction
has been changed by the retouching—there
are no composites.

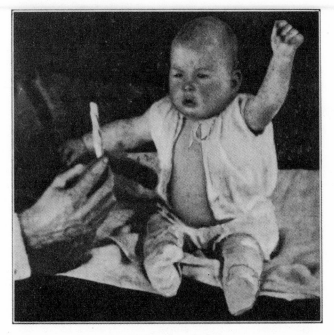

A test for handedness

Is handedness inherited or is it acquired? To test this we take the time infants can support themselves on a small stick first with right and then left hand. In older infants we hold out a stick of red candy. He reaches out with one or the other hand.

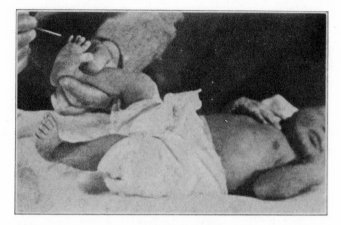

The Babinski Reflex

Here is a curious reaction in the new born. If the skin of the bottom of the foot is stroked, the toes fan out and the great toe flies upward (extension). When the foot of the adult is stroked sharply with the end of a match stick, all of the toes "clinch" or "grasp." In certain diseases of the nervous system the toes of the adult behave as do the toes of the child. This reaction, which in the child is due to the immaturity of the nervous system (not disease), disappears somewhere between the first and second years.

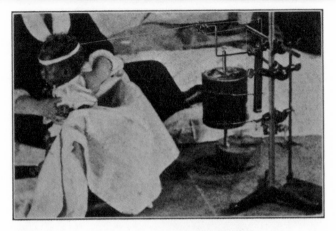

A test for head steadiness

At six months of age the infant should be able to hold up its head. To study the accuracy with which the head is held we place a soft band around the head of the child. Next we run a cord from this band to a lever which writes upon a smoked drum. If the head is held steady, the lever traces a straight line. Any wobbling of the head causes the lever to trace a wavy line. The photograph shows that this child at six months could hold its head fairly steady for several minutes.

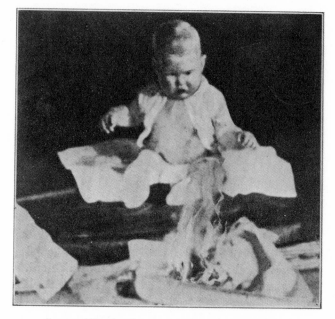

Intrepidly he faces fire for the first time

This child was kept under daily observation for nine months. He had never seen fire until posed for this photograph. He is looking at a lively fire made from newspapers. He shows not the slightest signs of fear.

This is one of a series of tests made to find out what children are afraid of apart from training or habit.

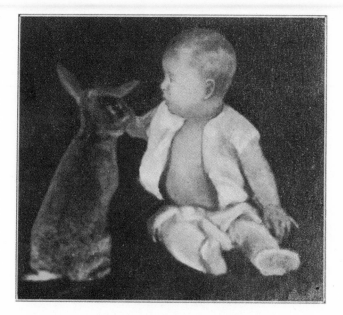

His first view of a rabbit

A great many people believe that children fear furry animals. This eight months old youngster is seeing a live, furry animal for the first time. He reaches for the rabbit as boldly as he reaches for his toys. Nor does he shudder and draw back when his hands touch the animal.

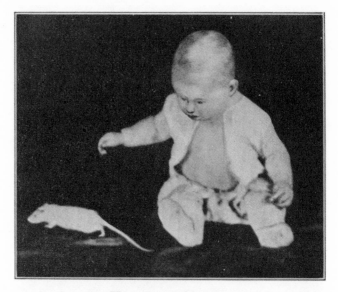

He sees a white rat

Additional proof that there is no fear of furry animals. This same youngster sees a white rat for the first time. He is reaching for it as fast as he can. Now most adults (especially women) are afraid of rats, but our work shows that all of these fears are *acquired*. We explain how on page 52.

Our tests on this and other children prove, we believe, conclusively that there is no inherited fear of furry animals.

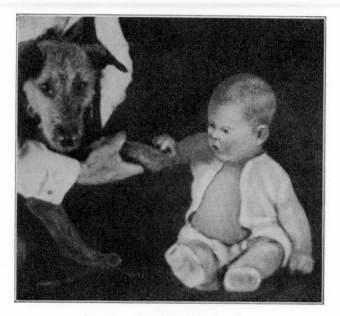

Shaking hands with the dog

There is a tradition that children are born afraid of large animals. Here is a large, *furry* Airedale many times the size of the baby. He is seeing it for the first time in his life. He promptly reaches out and begins to grasp its paws. No sign of fear is shown. Even when monkeys are shown him for the first time he reacts positively to them.

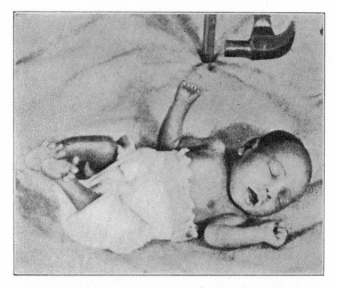

One thing he is afraid of

Our tests show that there are two things even the new born infant is afraid of and only two. One is shown above. The baby lies quietly on his blanket. A steel bar is struck with a hammer near his head. There is a start—a tensing of the muscles and then the cry. Many kinds of loud noises will produce this reaction—the banging of pans—a window shade racing upward—the fall of a screen or window.

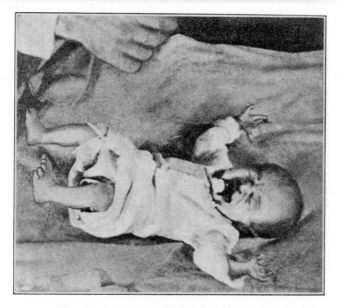

Loss of support his only other fear

The other thing the infant fears from birth is loss of support. The baby is shown here just after the blanket upon which he is lying is suddenly jerked. He cries and shows fear even if a "pacifier" is left in his mouth.

Our conclusions are that the human infant shows fear only in the presence of loud, sharp sounds and when *support* or *balance* is suddenly disturbed.

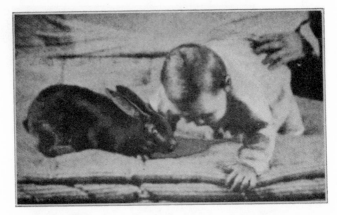

He now fears his furry friend

We see here a man-made, built in fear. This is the same infant shown playing with the rabbit on page 23. This fear was experimentally built in by the process of conditioning described on page 51. Now the moment the child sees the rabbit he cries, falls down and starts to crawl away.

Most of our fears are built in at an early age by happenings of one kind or another in the home and playground. Some practical suggestions for bringing a child up relatively free of fears grow out of these experiments. See page 60.

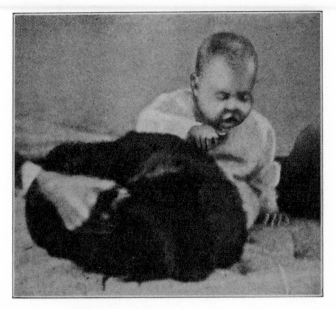

He runs away from a fur muff

After having been "conditioned" to fear the furry rabbit here is his reaction to a fur muff—seen for the first time. He now fears everything in the furry kingdom—dog, cat, rat, and rabbit, even fur muffs and neckpieces.

To fear these things he does not have to be separately conditioned on each one.

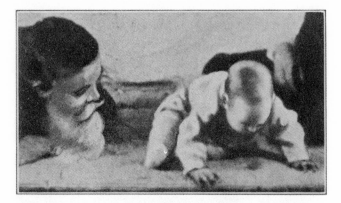

Now he fears even Santa Claus

After conditioning even the *sight* of the long whiskers of a Santa Claus mask sends the youngster scuttling away, crying and shaking his head from side to side. He had never seen a Santa Claus before. This reaction is also a direct result of our setting up in him conditioned fear of the rabbit.

After showing that fears can be built in experimentally, we next began work upon a way of removing them. We learned that they can be removed by a very simple common sense method. See p. 60.

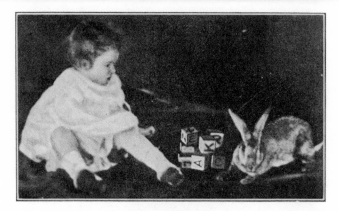

A home grown fear

Not all of the fears you see displayed are products of the laboratory. Here is a beautiful two and a half year old child, tenderly nurtured in one of our best American homes. She was frightened in infancy by a large dog when he jumped up on her carriage and barked in her ear. This one experience so conditioned her that she showed fear in the presence of dogs, rabbits, rats and monkeys.

This shows that when conditioning occurs in infancy the fear persists for a long period of time—possibly for life.

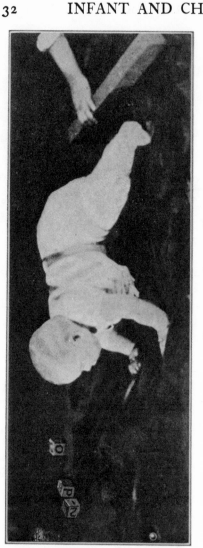

One to make ready

Another activity studied is how infants learn to crawl. The nine months old infant is shown here *coiled* to make a spring for the bright steel ball in front of him. A bar of wood marks his starting point. The photograph on the next page shows the completion of the act.

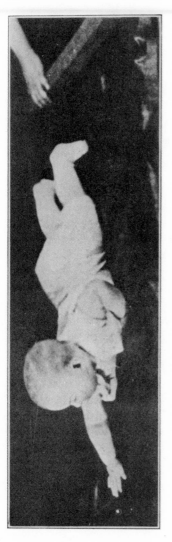

Three to go

This child, it can be seen, learned to crawl by coiling up on his knees as shown in the preceding photograph and then springing forward.

No two children learn to crawl in the same way. Some crawl by hitching along on one elbow, some by digging in the toes and pushing the body forward. Some infants practically never crawl. They learn to pull themselves upward by the help of some support and then pass from object to object.

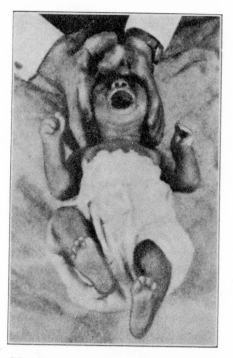

Holding the infant calls out rage

The one situation which from birth will call out the response of rage is interference with the infant's activity. Holding the head, legs or trunk gently but firmly will almost invariably call it out. Other objects come to call it out through conditioning—see page 96.

These tests are taken quite at random just to make clear what we are doing in the laboratory. We are testing literally hundreds of such infant responses. Let me enumerate a few more. Does the infant smell during the first week; does it hear; does it weep? How soon can it turn over, crawl, begin to form habits, use its thumb, blink when you pass your hand across its face? When does it make its first sound, when can you make it say its first word, when does it begin to play?

Why we make these tests

Why do we make these tests? To see what we have to start with—what we have to build upon to make a human being. To find a way of checking how our baby is getting on in its general development. To determine what a normal baby should do at birth, what it should be doing at one month—three months—six months—one year.

To give any real picture of our results and

of the methods used in studying child development would require time and patience beyond your present limits. After all, as parents we are interested more in what the behaviorist has found out and what he wants us "to do about it," than in the details of his work.

Some of the things we learn from these tests

When we first look at what the child can do at birth and soon thereafter, we are apt to be startled by the many things it can do rather than by those it cannot do. But the truth of the matter is that we find very little to wonder at in the birth equipment of the human child. Having studied both the newborn monkey and the newborn child in the laboratory, we now know that the newborn monkey can do everything the human infant can do and many, many other things beside. At one month of age the monkey infant can perform many acts of skill that the human child cannot do until many years have passed.

But to return to the child and its birth equipment. Even the simple reflexes we have just examined, such as breathing, the movement of the hands, arms, legs, trunk, smiling and crying, soon show the effect of your training—soon become influenced by the kind of life you force your child to lead. What it smiles at, what it cries about, what makes it catch its breath, what makes its heart beat slower or faster, depends in large measure upon the daily happenings in your home.

But you may ask, aren't there more complex inherited forms of behavior which appear later as *instincts?* Aren't such activities as *climbing, imitation, emulation* and *rivalry, pugnacity, anger, resentment, sympathy, hunting, fear, appropriation, acquisitiveness, kleptomania, constructiveness, play, curiosity, sociability, shyness, cleanliness, modesty, shame, love, jealousy, parental love,* pure instincts which appear and run their course completely beyond the control of the parents? Surely these things are not dependent upon the way I let my child grow up. Most of the older psychologists would agree with you. The behaviorist believed, too, when he began his work, that some of these acts would spring forth fully formed. But we waited for their appearance in vain. Now we are forced to believe from the study of facts that all of these forms of behavior are *built in* by the parent and by the environment which the parent allows the child to grow up in. There are no instincts. We build in at an early age everything that is later to appear.

Possibly we can better describe all this by saying that parents *slant* their children in age-old ways that reflect the way their own parents brought them up. If you take a young plant and put it near a lighted window, it bends toward the light. You slant the plant by putting it in a certain environment. If you grow an oak seedling out in the open and tie a weight to its tip, the shoot will begin to curve and grow downward. Just as surely do parents slant their children from the very moment of birth, nor does the slanting process ever end. The old, threadbare adage, "As the twig is bent so is the tree inclined," takes on a fresh meaning. You daily slant your children; you continue the process until they leave you. Even after they leave the home and your immediate influence, your slanting does not cease to exert its effect. It has become so fixed in their modes of behavior and even in their very thoughts that nothing can ever wholly eradicate it. Truly do we inevitably create our young in our own image.

Apply this to your child's vocational future. The vocation your child is to follow in later life is not determined from within, but from without—by you—by the kind of life you have made him lead. If he has no bent toward any vocation, the reason is equally due to your method of handling him. In a few cases where the child is physically defective, certain vocations become impossible, but these are so rarely met with that they need not influence our general conclusions.

This doctrine is almost the opposite of what is taught in the schools at the present time. Professor John Dewey and many other educators have been insisting for the last twenty years upon a method of training which allows the child to develop from within. This is really a doctrine of mystery. It teaches that there are hidden springs of activity, hidden possibilities of unfolding within the child which must be waited for until they appear and then be fostered and tended. I think this doctrine has done serious harm. It has made us lose our opportunity to implant and then to encourage a real eagerness for vocations at an early age. Some few thousands of undergraduates have passed through my hands. Only in the rarest of cases have I found a senior college student with his mind made up as to what vocation he will enter when he leaves college. There is no white heat for a certain type of career and no organization developed for seeing that career through. The young graduate today is almost as helpless as the straw tossed by the wind. He will take any kind of a job that chance may offer him in the hope that his special bents and aptitudes will show themselves. There is no reason why he shouldn't pick out his career at the age of 12 or earlier.

The behaviorists believe that there is nothing from within to develop. If you start with a healthy body, the right number of fingers and toes, eyes, and the few elementary movements that are present at birth, you do not need anything else in the way of raw material to make a man, be that man a genius, a cultured gentleman, a rowdy or a thug.

So much for general behavior, the behavior that you can directly observe in your children. But how about the things you cannot observe? How about *capacity, talent, temperament, personality,* "mental" constitution and "mental" characteristics, and the whole inward emotional life?

Let us take fear and timidity for a moment. We saw just now (pp. 26–27) that the only thing the child is afraid of at birth is either a loud sound or the loss of support. Everything else the child may fear is built in, is the result of the environment we let him grow up in. Until you have studied how all this comes about no one could expect you to know that you are completely responsible for all the other fear reactions your child may show. Does he avoid dark rooms, animals, strange people, strange situations? Is he timid and shy? Have you handicapped his whole future by making him shun new situations and new people?

How about temper, anger, rage? Only one simple situation will call out temper, anger, rage, namely, *restraint of the child's movements,* holding its arms and legs (p. 34). Temper and rage displayed in any other situation is home made. Parents do not realize that when they or their nurses are dressing their child badly, putting it in tight clothes, teasing it by holding its hands, or putting it in narrow quarters for punishment, they are organizing it in such a way that it will show throughout its life fits of anger and temper tantrums. A calmer mode of behavior would enable the child, and the adult it is to become, to conquer the environment instead of being overwhelmingly conquered by it.

How about its loves—its affectionate behavior? Isn't that "natural"? Do you mean to say the child doesn't *"instinctively"* love its mother? Only one thing will bring out a love response in the child—stroking and touching its skin, lips, sex organs and the like. It doesn't matter at first who strokes it. It will "love" the stroker. This is the clay out of which all love—maternal, paternal, wifely or husbandly—is made. Hard to believe? But true. A certain amount of affectionate response is socially necessary but few parents realize how easily they can overtrain the child in this direction. It may tear the heart strings a bit, this thought of stopping the tender outward demonstration of your love for your children or of their love for you. But if you are convinced that this is best for the child, aren't you willing to stifle a few pangs? Mothers just don't know, when they kiss their children and pick them up and rock them, caress them and jiggle them upon their knee, that they are slowly building up a human being totally unable to cope with the world it must later live in.

The various steps by which this building in process or *slanting* takes place in infancy are now fairly well known. Some of the steps can be actually watched in the laboratory. I hope to give you convincing proof of the accuracy of these facts in the following pages.

CHAPTER TWO

THE FEARS OF CHILDREN AND HOW TO
CONTROL THEM

CHILDREN'S fears are home grown just like their loves and temper outbursts. The parents do the emotional planting and the cultivating. At three years of age the child's whole emotional life plan has been laid down, his emotional disposition set. At that age the parents have already determined for him whether he is to grow into a happy person, wholesome and good-natured, whether he is to be a whining, complaining neurotic, an anger driven, vindictive, over-bearing slave driver, or one whose every move in life is definitely controlled by fear.

But how do parents build in fears?

In the preceding chapter I brought out the fact that all we have to start with in building a human being is a lively squirming bit of flesh, capable of making a few simple responses such as movements of the hands and arms and fingers and toes, crying and smiling, making certain sounds with its throat. I said there that parents take this raw material and begin to fashion it in ways to suit themselves. This means that parents, whether they know it or not, start intensive training of the child at birth.

It is especially easy to shape the emotional life at this early age. I might make this simple comparison: The fabricator of metal takes his heated mass, places it upon the anvil and begins to shape it according to patterns of his own. Sometimes he uses a heavy hammer, sometimes a light one; sometimes he strikes the yielding mass a mighty blow, sometimes he gives it just a touch. So inevitably do we begin at birth to shape the emotional life of our children. The blacksmith has all the advantage. If his strokes have been heavy and awkward and he spoils his work, he can put the metal back on the fire and start the process over. There is no way of starting over again with the child. Every stroke, be it true or false, has its effect. The best we can do is to conceal, skillfully as we may, the defects of our shaping. We can still make a useful instrument, an instrument that will work, but how few human instruments have ever been perfectly shaped to fit the environments in which they must function!

I think I can take you into the laboratory and give you a clear picture of the kinds of sledge hammers you are using in fashioning the fear life of your child.

Our laboratory work shows the fear life of the newborn infant is simplicity itself. From birth the child will show fear whenever a sudden loud sound is made close to its head and whenever it is thrown off its balance, as for example, when its blanket is quickly jerked (see page 27). No other fears are natural, all other fears are built in.

And yet, think how complicated is the fear

life of the three-year-old, the adolescent, the timid adult. Study the fears of the adults around you. I have seen a grown man cower and cringe and literally blanch with fear at the sight of a gun. I have seen a man stay all night in a hotel rather than enter his dark home when family and servants are away. I have seen a woman go into hysterics when a bat flew into a room. I have seen a child so torn by fear of moving animal toys that his whole organized life was in danger. Think of our fear of lightning, wind, railway trains, automobile accidents, ocean travel, burglars, fire, electricity and the thousands of other things that literally torture us even in this modern, supposedly secure life we lead. Think how peaceful, how calm, how efficient our lives would be if we were no more fearful than the newborn baby.

What can the laboratory say about the way fears grow up?

Suppose I put before you a beautiful,

healthy, well-formed baby nine months of age. On his mattress I place a rabbit. I know this baby's history; I know he has never seen a rabbit before. He reaches for the rabbit first with one hand, then the other the moment his eyes light upon it (p. 23). I replace the rabbit with a dog (p. 25). He behaves the same way. I next show him a cat, then a pigeon. Each new object is gleefully welcomed and equally gleefully handled. Afraid of furry objects? Not at all. But how about slimy objects? Surely he is afraid of cold, clammy, squirmy animals. Surely he is afraid of fish and frogs. I hand him a gold fish, alive and squirming. I put a green frog in front of him. Something new, again for the first time. Yes, a new world to work at. Immediately he goes after it as vigorously as after the other members of the animal kingdom. But surely all ancient history tells us that man instinctively avoids the snake. Literature is full of references to the fact that man's natural enemy is the snake. Not so with our lusty nine months infant.

The boa constrictor I put in front of him—when young the most harmless of snakes—calls out the most vigorous of all those favorable friendly responses.

But won't our infant cry out in fear when I put him in the total darkness of a light-proof room? Not at all. But won't flame, that most terrifying of all physical agents, when seen for the first time at this tender age throw him almost into a fit? Let us take an iron pan and make a little bonfire of newspapers, being careful to keep it far enough away to keep the child from harm (p. 22).

This infant must be phlegmatic, without emotional life. Not at all. I can convince you easily otherwise. In my hands I have a steel bar about an inch in diameter and about four feet long, and a carpenter's hammer (see page 26 for this test on the newborn). The child is sitting up looking at the attendant. I hold the steel bar about a foot behind his head where he can't see me. I rap the steel bar sharply with the hammer. The picture changes immediately. First a whimper, a sudden catching of the breath, a stiffening of the whole body, a pulling of the hands to the side, then a cry, then tears. I bang it again. The reaction becomes still more pronounced. He cries out loud, rolls over to his side and begins to crawl away as rapidly as possible.

Suppose I let him sit quietly on a blanket over his mattress. He may be very still, just dozing, or he may be playing eagerly with a toy. Suddenly I jerk the blanket, pull his support from under him. This sudden loss of support produces almost the same reaction as the loud sound (see p. 27 for this test on the newborn). I haven't hurt him by pulling the blanket, he falls over from his sitting position fifty times a day and never whimpers. Your training has nothing to do with the fear he shows at loud sounds and loss of support, nor will any training ever completely remove the potency of these things to call out fears. I have seen the most seasoned hunter when dozing, jump violently when his comrade strikes a match to kindle the camp fire. You have seen the most intrepid of women show terror in crossing a perfectly safe foot bridge that sways with her weight.

Fear of all other objects is home-made. Now to prove it. Again I put in front of you the nine months old infant. I have my assistant take his old playmate, the rabbit, out of its pasteboard box and hand it to him. He starts to reach for it. But just as his hands touch it I bang the steel bar behind his head. He whimpers and cries and shows fear. Then I wait awhile. I give him his blocks to play with. He quiets down and soon becomes busy with them. Again my assistant shows him the rabbit. This time he reacts to it quite slowly. He doesn't plunge his hands out as quickly and eagerly as before. Finally he does touch it gingerly. Again I strike the steel bar behind his head. Again I get a pronounced fear response. Then I let him quiet down. He plays with his blocks. Again the assistant brings in the rabbit. This time something new develops.

No longer do I have to rap the steel bar behind his head to bring out fear. *He shows fear at the sight of the rabbit.* He makes the same reaction to it that he makes to the sound of the steel bar. He begins to cry and turn away the moment he sees it (p. 28).

I have started the process of fear building. And this fear of the rabbit persists. If you show the rabbit to him one month later, you get the same reaction. There is good evidence to show that such early built in fears last throughout the lifetime of the individual.

We have a name in the laboratory for fears built up in this experimental way. We call them *conditioned* fears and we mean by that "home-made fears." By this method we can, so far as we know, make any object in the world call out a *conditioned* fear response. All we have to do is to show the infant any object and make a loud sound at the same moment.

But this fear of the rabbit is not the only building stone we have laid in the child's life of fear. After this one experience, and with no further contact with animals, all furry animals such as the dog, the cat, the rat, the guinea pig, may one and all call out fear. He becomes afraid even of a fur coat, a rug or a Santa Claus mask. He does not have to touch them; just seeing them will call out fear. (p. 28 ff.) This simple experiment gives us a startling insight into the ways in which our early home surroundings can build up fears. You may think that such experiments are cruel, but they are not cruel if they help us to understand the fear life of the millions of people around us and give us practical help in bringing up our children more nearly free from fears than we ourselves have been brought up. They will be worth all they cost if through them we can find a method which will help us remove fear.

How we build up fears in the home

But, you say, these are laboratory experiments. What have they to do with the home?

How do the parents build in these fears? In the simplest kinds of ways. Just think of the noises in the home; and the younger the child, the less organized it is, the more likely are these noises to produce fear reactions. Let me enumerate a few of them. Your child has shown a little unwillingness to go to bed. This has hampered your own movements a bit and you slam the door when you go out. You want your child to live in a well ventilated room; you open all the windows on a breezy night. Before you get to the door, it slams. In the night when the child is sleeping soundly the shade falls down or the screen placed around its crib falls over. Doors slam all over the house on windy nights, pots and pans are dropped. All of these things are powerful agents, they are sledge hammers in the shaping of your child. No flash of lightning can ever scare your child; even a beam of bright sunlight flashed upon its face in its darkened room will cause only a squinting of the eye. But the loud sizzling crack of thunder overhead will call out a scream of terror and thereafter the flash of lightning may call out the most pronounced fit of terror. If the child happens to be in a darkened room when the peal of thunder occurs it may become afraid of the dark for days and weeks.

Another type of behavior to be closely watched

Another part of the child's behavior closely connected with its fear life must be carefully watched by the parents. Whenever the child's body is being injured, as happens when pin pricks, burns, pinching and slapping occur, a negative or withdrawal reaction takes place. Every infant is born with the ability to withdraw any part of its body from the object that is injuring it. These reactions are sometimes called *avoidance* reactions. An easy way to express all this is to say that the child jerks its hand away from a painful object, a burn or a slap, for example. All negative reactions except those coming from painful objects are home-made or built in by the parents. Most of us have thousands of these negative reactions built in. We avoid places, things, people. Negative or withdrawal reactions are *conditioned* just as are our reactions to fear. Let me illustrate. The crawling child reaches out and touches the hot radiator. It jerks its hand back. Sometimes one such experience is enough to keep the child three feet away from that object. After it has been negatively conditioned to radiators, the mere sight of a radiator makes the infant pull its hand away.

The parents' "don't" is a mighty sledge hammer

The parents' "don't" is the most potent factor of all in producing both fear and negative responses. Have you as a parent ever stopped to consider how many times a day you use "don't"? Do you know that when you use it you are using a mighty sledge hammer for molding fear and other negative reactions in your child?

Now the simple word "don't" has no power in itself to produce either a negative or a fear reaction in the child. It must borrow this power. Where does it get it? In two ways. The father has a powerful voice. Just at the moment the child starts to reach for something or to perform some act not desired by the father, he yells "Don't!" You have everything ready to produce a conditioned fear reaction. The powerful word "don't" takes the place of the steel bar in our laboratory experiment. In a short time the child shows a fear reaction when in that situation. "Don't" derives its sledge hammer power in another way. Often when the child reaches for an object one of the parents slaps its fingers and says "don't" at the same time. Now the slapping or painful stimulus will make the child jerk back its hand. Again we have a situation at hand for setting up a conditioned negative response. "Don't" soon takes on the same power to produce fear and negative reactions as loud sounds and painful objects. Because of the frequency with which we use them, "don't" and words like it soon become the ruling forces in the life of every child. The power of the state, church and society is built upon this simple principle. They all teach us to live a life of fear. I quarrel with them not as institutions but because of their methods of instruction. In a similar way, hundreds of other words and sentences take on the same powerful significance. Even as adults we feel the potency of: "Don't touch that dog, it will bite you!" "That thing might explode!" "The match will burn you up!" "Don't touch fire, it is hot!" "That water is deep—there is a heavy undertow!" The terms "wicked", "wrong", "sin", "pirate", "enemy", "the devil", "Satan", all get their reaction-producing effects in this simple way.

*Simple things parents can do to keep their
children freer from fears and negative
reactions*

Should we have no noise in the house where
a baby is growing up? Should the parents'
lives become a burden? Should they have to
tiptoe around the house day and night in order
to avoid setting up conditioned fear responses?
There is not the slightest psychological reason
for this. Only loud sudden noises of a certain
character will produce these negative reactions. Hence the home life can go on in its
normal way without regard to sleeping or
waking infants. Why shouldn't the piano be
played, the radio, the phonograph? Why
shouldn't people dance and walk and talk
around the house naturally? The child
brought up with normal noises around it is
never later disturbed by them unless it is ill,
in which case the normal noise should be
started again as soon as it gets well.

Parents can enormously lessen the possibility of loud sudden sounds occurring in the house. Doors should carefully be kept from slamming, shades should be securely fastened, screens should be placed so they cannot fall over. When a wind comes up suddenly the room should be looked over to prevent sudden noises. Of course, few of us have ideal homes for raising children. To start with our houses should be set far enough back from the roads to keep out explosions from automobiles, the loud honking of horns, the sharp barking of dogs. Even then thunder storms would be entirely out of our control!

Again the child should be carefully guarded from objects which will prick, burn or otherwise injure its skin. I think most parents are careful about this. Diapers are one of the most frequent causes of these negative reactions which produce crying and broken sleep, if they are put on so as to cause painful constriction, or with a pin not securely closed, or if they are left on when the skin has been allowed to chap or otherwise become sore.

Our slaps should be used as sparingly as possible, too. So also the word "don't", which is the equivalent of the slap.

Should no fear reactions be built in—should we never say "don't" and never slap?

I think some fears and other negative responses should be built in. If the child is going to get along in the group it is later to be thrown into, a certain kind of conformity with group standards must be established. I do not hesitate when children begin reaching for objects not their own to rap their fingers smartly, with a pencil. To get the right psychological conditions, the parent should always apply this painful stimulus just at the moment the undesirable act is taking place. If you wait for father to spank when he gets home it is practically impossible to establish a conditioned negative response. Unless negatively conditioned in this way how else will children learn not to reach for glasses and vases? How can they learn not to touch strange dogs, fondle strange cats, to walk out into the water? But the building in of these necessary negative responses and gentler fear responses, both by the word "don't" and by rapping the fingers smartly, must not be looked upon as punishing the child in the old sense. The word punishment should not appear in our dictionaries except as an obsolete word, and I believe this should be just as true in the field of criminology as in that of child rearing. The parents' object in rapping the child with a pencil is to get it to react in conformity with certain social usages—to behave itself. Why then should the parents ever be angry? Why should they ever punish in the old biblical sense? Such things as beating and expiation of offences, so common now in our schools and homes, in the church, in our criminal law, in our judicial procedure, are relics of the Dark Ages. The parents' attitude should be positive, should be that of the instructor. We can sum it all up by saying that the behaviorist advocates the early building in of appropriate common sense negative reactions by the method of gently rapping the fingers or hand or other bodily part when the undesirable act is taking place, *but as an objective experimental procedure*—never as punishment.

So that we can cut down the number of negative reactions we have to build in, we should keep the child in an environment where its reactions can be positive. We should keep it busy during the day doing things instead of not doing things. By surrounding the child constantly with objects that it can build up and manipulate, we soon get it to form habits of working with objects that it has a right to work with. In this way "forbidden" objects come gradually to lose their stimulating value; the children cease to play with fire, with matches, they stop turning gas jets on and off, picking up sharp knives and forks, pulling over glass vases and bottles. But where the positive method of training does not make them let these objects alone, then gentle pencil rapping is a safe and sane procedure.

How can we remove fear of objects which should not be feared?

But fears do get built in no matter how careful we are. Can we remove them?

It is difficult to remove fears. It requires patience. It requires an experimental attitude on the part of the parent. Suppose your child shows a deep-seated fear of a rabbit. You can keep the rabbit away indefinitely but when you show it a year later the chances are good that the fear will again show itself. Just keeping the fearsome object away (disuse) will not effect a cure.

You can try reading stories about the rabbit to your child—organizing its verbal life ("reasoning") about the rabbit. This will not cure the fear.

You can try ridicule—call him " 'fraidy

cat," etc.—but without result. You will only complicate his emotional life.

You can try letting other children play with the rabbit in front of the scared child. This does not work either.

When all other methods fail, try this method which was developed in the laboratory by Mrs. Mary Cover Jones. Work it only once per day, at noontime, when the child is hungry. Just as the child sees its food, let some one show the rabbit as far away as possible. You may have to open the hall door if the dining room is not large enough to get the rabbit far enough away. When the rabbit is far enough away the child will begin to eat. Do not let it ever see the rabbit except at this one time during the day. The next day when the child begins to eat show the rabbit first at the same point where it was shown the day before. Then bring it a little nearer. When the child begins to show fear stop the advance. Repeat this procedure every day. Soon the child can tolerate the *rabbit on the table*, then in its lap. Tranquillity descends; the fear is gone permanently. We call this process *un-conditioning*. Retraining by this method has a widespread effect. It removes the fear of other furry animals, or at least greatly modifies it.

Suppose your child has suddenly been made afraid of the dark, don't rave and storm at it. Start unconditioning at once. Put the child to bed at its usual time. Leave a faint light in the hall and leave the door open. Then every night after putting the child to bed close the door a little more and dim the light still more. Three or four nights usually suffice.

Suppose your child has lost its balance in the water or has been made negative to its bath by slipping and falling so that the morning bath becomes a terror—not an unusual thing. Don't take the child to the bathroom for a time. Give it a sponge bath in the nursery for a day or two; then use a wash basin with a little water in it. Increase the water in the basin. Begin to use a wetter sponge. In a few days you can take the child back again to its regular bath. I have seen fathers especially almost ruin their children's chances of learning to swim and dive by forcing them into the water.

Just ordinary *common sense*—this helps us to prevent fears in the home. By unconditioning as soon as fear of any object did develop, I have seen several sets of children grow up practically without fear of animals (although they would not touch strange ones), without fear, timidity or shyness in the presence of strangers, without fear of the dark, fire or any other object animate or inanimate. Fear behavior can be taught just as easily as reading and writing, building with blocks or drawing. It can be taught well or badly. When taught scientifically the emotional life is then under "control."

Surely every mother with a timid, fearful child will be more than willing, now that she knows how to start, to take the time and trouble necessary sensibly to shape the fear life of her child.

CHAPTER THREE

THE DANGERS OF TOO MUCH MOTHER LOVE

ONCE at the close of a lecture before parents, a dear old lady got up and said, "Thank God, my children are grown—and that I had a chance to enjoy them before I met you."

Doesn't she express here the weakness in our modern way of bringing up children? We have children to enjoy them. We need to express our love in some way. The honeymoon period doesn't last forever with all husbands and wives, and we eke it out in a way we think is harmless by loving our children to death. Isn't this especially true of the mother today? No matter how much she may love her husband, he is away all day; her heart is full of love which she must express in some way. She expresses it by showering love and kisses upon

69

her children—and thinks the world should laud her for it. *And it does.*

Not long ago, I went motoring with two boys, aged four and two, their mother, grandmother and nurse. In the course of the two-hour ride, one of the children was kissed thirty-two times—four by his mother, eight by the nurse and twenty times by the grandmother. The other child was almost equally smothered in love.

But there are not many mothers like that, you say—mothers are getting modern, they do not kiss and fondle their children nearly so much as they used to. Unfortunately this is not true. I once let slip in a lecture some of my ideas on the dangers lurking in the mother's kiss. Immediately, thousands of newspapers wrote scathing editorials on "Don't kiss the baby." Hundreds of letters poured in. Judging from them, kissing the baby to death is just about as popular a sport as it ever was, except for a very small part of our population.

Is it just the hard heartedness of the behaviorist—his lack of sentiment—that makes
him object to kissing? Not at all. There are
serious rocks ahead for the over-kissed child.
Before I name them I want to explain how
love grows up.

Our laboratory studies show that we can
bring out a love response in a newborn child
by just one stimulus—*by stroking its skin*. The
more sensitive the skin area, the more marked
the response. These sensitive areas are the
lips, ears, back of the neck, nipples and the sex
organs. If the child is crying, stroking these
areas will often cause the child to become
quiet or even to smile. Nurses and mothers
have learned this method of quieting an infant by the trial and error process. They pick
the child up, pat it, scothe it, kiss it, rock it,
walk with it, dandle it on the knee, and the
like. All of this kind of petting has the result of gently stimulating the skin. Unscru-
pulous nurses have learned the very direct
result which comes from stroking the sex or-

gans. When the child gets older, the fondling, petting, patting, rocking of the body will bring out a gurgle or a coo, open laughter, and extension of the arms for the embrace.

The love life of the child is *at birth* very simple as is all of its other emotional behavior. Touching and stroking of the skin of the young infant brings out a love response. No other stimulus will.

This means that there is no "instinctive" love of the child for the parents, nor for any other person or object. It means that all affection, be it parental, child for parent or love between the sexes, is built up with such bricks and mortar. A great many parents who have much too much sentiment in their make-up, feel that when the behaviorist announces this he is robbing them of all the sacredness and sweetness in the child-parent relationship. Parents feel that it is just natural that they should love their children in this tangible way and that they should be similarly loved by the child in return. Some of the most tor-

tured moments come when the parents have
had to be away from their nine-months old
baby for a stretch of three weeks. When they
part from it, the child gurgles, coos, holds
out its arms and shows every evidence of deepest parental love. Three weeks later when they
return the child turns to the attendant who has
in the interim fondled and petted it and put
the bottle to the sensitive lips. The infant child
loves anyone who strokes and feeds it.

It is true that parents have got away from
rocking their children to sleep. You find the
cradle with rockers on it now only in exhibits
of early American furniture. You will say
that we have made progress in this respect
at any rate. This is true. Dr. Holt's book on
the care of the infant can take credit for this
education. But it is doubtful if mothers would
have given it up if home economics had not
demanded it. Mothers found that if they
started training the infant at birth, it would
learn to go to sleep without rocking. This
gave the mother more time for household

duties, gossiping, bridge and shopping. Dr. Holt suggested it; the economic value of the system was easy to recognize.

But it doesn't take much time to pet and kiss the baby. You can do it when you pick him up from the crib after a nap, when you put him to bed, and especially after his bath. What more delectable to the mother than to kiss her chubby baby from head to foot after the bath! And it takes so little time!

To come back to the mechanics of love and affection. Loves grow up in children just like fears. *Loves* are home made, built in. In other words loves are *conditioned*. You have everything at hand all day long for setting up conditioned love responses. The touch of the skin takes the place of the steel bar, the sight of the mother's face takes the place of the rabbit in the experiments with fear. The child *sees* the mother's face when she pets it. Soon, *the mere sight of the mother's face* calls out the love response. The touch of the skin is no longer necessary to call it out. A conditioned love reaction has been formed. Even if she pats the child in the dark, the *sound* of her voice as she croons soon comes to call out a love response. This is the psychological explanation of the child's joyous reactions to the sound of the mother's voice. So with her footsteps, the sight of the mother's clothes, of her photograph. All too soon the child gets shot through with too many of these love reactions. In addition the child gets honeycombed with love responses for the nurse, for the father and for any other constant attendant who fondles it. Love reactions soon dominate the child. It requires no instinct, no "intelligence," no "reasoning" on the child's part for such responses to grow up.

The adult effects of too much coddling in infancy

To understand the end results of too much coddling, let us examine some of our own adult behavior. Nearly all of us have suffered from over-coddling in our infancy. How does it show? It shows as *invalidism*. As adults we have too many aches and pains. I rarely ask anybody with whom I am constantly thrown how he feels or how he slept last night. Almost invariably, if I am a person he doesn't have to keep up a front around, I get the answer, "Not very well." If I give him the chance, he expatiates along one of the following lines—"my digestion is poor; I have a constant headache; my muscles ache like fire; I am all tired out; I don't feel young any more; my liver is bad; I have a bad taste in my mouth"—and so on through the whole gamut of ills. Now these people have nothing wrong with them that the doctors can locate —and with the wonderful technique physicians have developed, the doctor can usually find out if anything is wrong. The individual who was not taught in his youth by his mother to be dependent, is one who comes to adult life too busy with his work to note the tiny mishaps that occur in his bodily makeup.

When we are deeply engaged in our work, we never note them. Can you imagine an aviator flying in a fog or making a landing in a difficult field wondering whether his luncheon is going to digest?

We note these ills when our routine of work no longer thrills us. We have been taught from infancy to report every little ill, to talk about our stomach, our elimination processes, and the like. We have been allowed to avoid the doing of boresome duties by reporting them, such as staying away from school and getting relieved from sharing in the household chores. And above all, we have, by reporting them, got the tender solicitude of our parents and the kisses and coddling of our mothers. Mother fights our battles for us and stands between us and the things we try to avoid doing.

But society doesn't do this. We have to stick to our jobs in commercial and professional life regardless of headaches, toothaches, indigestion and other tiny ailments. There is no one

there to baby us. If we cannot stand this treat-
ment we have to go back home where love
and affection can again be commandeered. If
at home we cannot get enough coddling by ordinary means, we take to our armchairs or
even to our beds. Thereafter we are in a secure
position to demand constant coddling.

You can see invalidism in the making in
the majority of American homes. Here is a
picture of a child over-conditioned in love.
The child is alone putting his blocks together,
doing something with his hands, learning how
to control his environment. The mother comes
in. Constructive play ceases. The child crawls
its way or runs to the mother, takes hold of
her, climbs into her lap, puts its arms around
her neck. The mother, nothing loath, fondles
her child, kisses it, hugs it. I have seen this go
on for a two-hour period. If the mother who
has so conditioned her child attempts to put
it down, a heartbroken wail ensues. Blocks
and the rest of the world have lost their pulling power. If the mother attempts to leave the

room or the house, a still more heartbroken cry ensues. Many mothers often sneak away from their homes the back way in order to avoid a tearful, wailing parting.

Now over-conditioning in love is the rule. Prove it yourself by counting the number of times your child whines and wails "Mother." All over the house, all day long, the two-year-old, the three-year-old and the four-year-old whine "Mamma, Mamma," "Mother." Now these love responses which the mother or father is building in by over conditioning, in spite of what the poet and the novelist may have to say, are not constructive. They do not fight many battles for the child. They do not help it to conquer the difficulties it must meet in its environment. Hence just to the extent to which you devote time to petting and coddling—and I have seen almost all of the child's waking hours devoted to it— just to that extent do you rob the child of the time which he should be devoting to the manipulation of his universe, acquiring a technique with fingers, hands and arms. He must have time to pull his universe apart and put it together again. Even from this standpoint alone—that of robbing the child of its opportunity for conquering the world, coddling is a dangerous experiment.

The mother coddles the child for two reasons. One, she admits; the other, she doesn't admit because she doesn't know that it is true. The one she admits is that she wants the child to be happy, she wants it to be surrounded by love in order that it may grow up to be a kindly, goodnatured child. The other is that her own whole being cries out for the expression of love. Her mother before her has trained her to give and receive love. She is starved for love—affection, as she prefers to call it. It is at bottom a sex-seeking response in her, else she would never kiss the child on the lips. Certainly, to satisfy her professed reason for coddling, kissing the youngster on the forehead, on the back of the hand, patting it on the head once in a while, would be all the petting needed for a baby to learn that it is growing up in a kindly home.

But even granting that the mother thinks she kisses the child for the perfectly logical reason of implanting the proper amount of affection and kindliness in it, does she succeed? The fact I brought out before, that we rarely see a happy child, is proof to the contrary. The fact that our children are always crying and always whining shows the unhappy, unwholesome state they are in. Their digestion is interfered with and probably their whole glandular system is deranged.

Should the mother never kiss the baby?

There is a sensible way of treating children. Treat them as though they were young adults. Dress them, bathe them with care and circumspection. Let your behavior always be objective and kindly firm. Never hug and kiss them, never let them sit in your lap. If you must, kiss them once on the forehead when they say good night. Shake hands with them in the morning. Give them a pat on the head if they have made an extraordinarily good job of a difficult task. Try it out. In a week's time you will find how easy it is to be perfectly objective with your child and at the same time kindly. You will be utterly ashamed of the mawkish, sentimental way you have been handling it.

If you expected a dog to grow up and be useful as a watch dog, a bird dog, a fox hound, useful for anything except a lap dog, you wouldn't dare treat it the way you treat your child. When I hear a mother say "Bless its little heart" when it falls down, or stubs its toe, or suffers some other ill, I usually have to walk a block or two to let off steam. Can't the mother train herself when something happens to the child to look at its hurt without saying anything, and if there is a wound to dress it in a matter of fact way? And then as the child grows older, can she not train it to go and find the boracic acid and the bandages and treat its own wounds? Can't she train herself to substitute a kindly word, a smile, in all of her dealings with the child, for the kiss and the hug, the pickup and coddling? Above all, can't she learn to keep away from the child a large part of the day since love conditioning must grow up anyway, even when scrupulously guarded against, through feeding and bathing? I sometimes wish that we could live in a community of homes where each home is supplied with a well-trained nurse so that we could have the babies fed and bathed each week by a different nurse. Not long ago I had opportunity to observe a child who had had an over sympathetic and tender nurse for a year and a half. This nurse had to leave. When a new nurse came, the infant cried for three hours, letting up now and then only long enough to get its breath. This nurse had to leave at the end of a month and a new nurse came. This time the infant cried only half an hour when the new nurse took charge of it. Again, as often happens in well regulated homes, the second nurse stayed only two weeks. When the third nurse came, the child went to her without a murmur. Somehow I can't help wishing that it were possible to rotate the mothers occasionally too! Unless they are very sensible indeed.

Certainly a mother, when necessary, ought to leave her child for a long enough period for over-conditioning to die down. If you haven't a nurse and cannot leave the child, put it out in the backyard a large part of the day. Build a fence around the yard so that you are sure no harm can come to it. Do this from the time it is born. When the child can crawl, give it a sandpile and be sure to dig some small holes in the yard so it has to crawl in and out of them. Let it learn to overcome difficulties almost from the moment of birth. The child should learn to conquer difficulties away from your watchful eye. No child should get commendation and notice and petting every time it does something it ought to be doing anyway. If your heart is too tender and you must watch the child, make yourself a peephole so that you can see it without being seen, or use a periscope. But above all when anything does happen don't let your child see your own trepidation, handle the situation as a trained nurse or a doctor would and, finally, learn not to talk in endearing and coddling terms.

Nest habits, which come from coddling, are really pernicious evils. The boys or girls who have nest habits deeply imbedded suffer torture when they have to leave home to go into business, to enter school, to get married—in general, whenever they have to break away from parents to start life on their own. Inability to break nest habits is probably our most prolific source of divorce and marital disagreements. "Mother's boy" has to talk his married life over with his mother and father, has constantly to bring them into the picture. The bride coddled in her infancy runs home to mother or father taking her trunk every time a disagreement occurs. We have hundreds of pathological cases on record where the mother or father attachment has become so strong that a marital adjustment even after marriage has taken place becomes impossible. To escape the intolerable marriage tie the individual becomes insane or else suicides. In the milder cases, though, the struggle between young married people coddled in infancy shows itself in whines and complaints and the endless recounting of ills. Not enjoying the activities that come with marriage they escape them by tiredness and headaches. If his wife does not give mother's boy the coddling, the commendation and the petting the mother gave him, she doesn't understand him, she is cold, unwifely, unsympathetic. If the young wife does not constantly receive the gentle coddling and admiration her father gave her then the husband is a brute, unsympathetic, un-understanding. Young married couples who do not swear a solemn oath to fight out their own battles between themselves without lugging in the parents soon come upon rocks.

In conclusion won't you then remember when you are tempted to pet your child that mother love is a dangerous instrument? An instrument which may inflict a never healing wound, a wound which may make infancy unhappy, adolescence a nightmare, an instrument which may wreck your adult son or daughter's vocational future and their chances for marital happiness.

CHAPTER FOUR

RAGE AND TEMPER TANTRUMS AND HOW TO CONTROL THEM

"MINE!" says Jimmy the two-year-old. "It isn't, it's mine; Mother, make Jimmy give me my harmonica," says Billy the four-year-old.

A fight ensues.

Billy wins out and Jimmy screams until he is black in the face.

Mother comes. She may try several different ways to straighten out the matter. Usually whatever she does is wrong. She may spank Billy for jerking the harmonica away from Jimmy, thus starting him off on a crying fit and a temper tantrum of his own, possibly sowing the first seeds of inferiority and cowardice in her older child. She may hug and kiss and pet the raging Jimmy, thus insuring rage behavior on his part the next time such a set-to occurs.

If she is a wise mother, she will have prepared herself in advance for just such a scene. When her children are so near together in age, she will have purchased identical toys for both boys. When a scene occurs she will go quietly and get the mate of the toy in question, take both the toys in her hands, show them and when crying stops offer them to the young hopefuls.

Neither youngster is to be blamed for the scene. It is perfectly natural for every young child to reach out for any object that catches his eye. Young children are positive,—i. e., reach for nearly all objects. Seeing the harmonica in Billy's hands, Jimmy reaches for it. It is only after we have suffered grief at the hands of mother, father, nurse or society for reaching out for forbidden objects that we come finally to withdraw our hands or our body from these objects. If, now, we could charge Billy's toys with electricity so that he could play with them with impunity but so arrange affairs that Jimmy would get shocked with the current whenever he reached for Billy's toys, then Jimmy would soon learn to keep his hands off Billy's toys. But in real nursery life toys cannot be charged with electricity. A row begins when the older (or stronger) boy forcibly takes something out of the hands of the younger boy, pushes his hands or shoves him. Note that the older boy does not actually hurt the younger (no pain stimulus is present) ; *he merely interferes with or hampers the movement of the younger.*

This stimulus, *hampering of movements,* will bring out a rage response even in the newborn. They do not have to learn to struggle when forcibly held. They squirm, kick and struggle at birth. In some of our first experiments upon the newborn infant we tried to find out whether it could turn its eyes towards a source of light without movement of the whole head. To test this we laid the child flat upon its back upon a mattress in a dark room. Immediately above its head we placed a very faint electric light. The light was arranged so that we could show it either to the right or the left of the infant's head. In order to keep the infant from turning its head, the experimenter held the head gently but firmly in his two hands. A soft cotton pad was placed on each side of the head so that the experimenter's hands did not come into direct contact with the scalp. Even when very little pressure was exerted upon the head the infant began to cry and, if we continued to hold its head, it went into a real fit of rage.

The same thing happens when we hold the feet or the legs together. In no case do we exert pressure enough to cause real pain. The response is first struggling, then crying. If the holding or hampering continues, the mouth opens wider and wider, the breath is held sometimes up to the point where not a sound can be heard, although the mouth is stretched to its fullest extent. The body grows rigid and the face becomes first flushed and then almost black. Here indeed is a new find in the laboratory. Rage or temper is a response which is

present in the newborn and its stimulus is
holding or hampering any part of the body.
In other words, the emotional situation is
quite similar to that of fear. In fear, you will
recall, only loud sounds and loss of support
will at first bring out the response. The photograph (p. 34) shows a newborn infant in a
rage fit and the stimulus which calls it out,
namely, holding the head.

Nor will any amount of training ever completely eliminate the rage response. Watch the
angry looks and fights which occur when
some rude person shoulders his way through
the crowd stepping upon toes and jostling the
arms of newspaper readers. Watch the struggles of an individual who is tied up or locked
up in a narrow closet. If you want an adult
demonstration of this primitive reaction, try
walking into a very crowded suburban car with
a heavy suitcase that jostles and rubs against
the people who are packed in around you.

In the newborn, temper is called out many
times every day,—in fact almost every time

we dress, undress, or change them, unless we handle them very smoothly and carefully and quickly. The present mode of dressing children seems eminently adapted to encourage rage behavior. After bathing them sometimes not too carefully from the standpoint of hampering them, we put a tight woolen band on them. Then somehow without actually wrenching their arms off, we put on a woolen shirt with sleeves. Next we roll them and twist them into a diaper and bundle them up so that their legs are never free for the first eighteen months (at night for a much longer time). Then by a highly developed system of gymnastics we get a woolen petticoat over the head; then usually a white petticoat next goes over the head—if the head is still there! Nor does it help much to start the other way—by poking their feet through first. Finally we pull and twist them into shoes. Then we tug and pull them into a sweater. If the baby is going out, it must be pulled into a cloth coat with sleeves. And as the baby gets a little stouter the woolen things get a little smaller because of their various trips to the laundry. The job of dressing becomes more and more of a gymnastic feat. Please understand that I am raising no quarrel with wool; it is very essential for the infant, so the medical authorities tell us. Nor have I very much to offer in the way of dress reform. I am merely bringing out the fact that dressing the infant with modern clothes gives us almost a laboratory set up for building in rage behavior.

So far we have talked only about the original stimulus to rage behavior. You will recall in previous chapters how fears and loves are built up in the home. Our experiments in the laboratory proved that almost unwittingly we make children fear more and more objects and show attachments for more and more people and things. We call this a process of *conditioning*. These new fears we call conditioned fears, the new loves conditioned loves.

Conditioned rages and tempers grow up in the same way. Here is a youngster in front of me whose movements I have interfered with from the day of his birth. In order to carry out a certain test upon him, I hold his hands until they begin to stiffen. I shake him a little, sometimes hold his nose. This brings out the grasping reflex in the hands. I then slip a tiny stick into his hands. He grasps it tightly. I lift him and let him support himself over a feather pillow. Just the instant he begins to release his hold my assistant catches him. Nearly always he goes into a rage the moment this test starts. After three or four such tests *the mere sight* of my face drove the youngster into a rage. *I no longer have to hamper his movement.* A conditioned rage response has been built in. After this experiment had been in progress twice weekly for two months, I tried to find out how close I could get to him without calling out this behavior. I found I couldn't get closer than eight to ten feet. At that distance the mere *sight* of my face was too much for him and the tantrum began. You see how simple it was to build in this behavior even in a newborn. The natural stimulus to his rage was the hampering of his movements when I forced him to grasp the stick, but *the youngster saw me as I hampered his movements.*

In this way apparently we can make any object call out rage. All we have to do is to show the object when we hamper the child's movements. Temper tantrums are thus built in by the thousands, just by ordinary daily happenings. This behavior we built into this child persisted as long as we had the child in the laboratory—and long after we had quit hampering his movements.

Does this experiment give you any insight into what goes on in your own home? Often nurses (and even mothers themselves) are a little impatient and, not realizing what they are doing, bathe the child hastily and carelessly, paw out its nose and ears, hold its legs apart while powdering, hold its arms down tightly to its sides while drying its body. Then they put it into its clothes almost ruthlessly.

The infant thus becomes conditioned not only on the paraphernalia of the bath but upon the person who does the bathing and dressing. Going to bed, getting dressed become signals for temper to begin. Often mothers who have learned to handle their children gently at the bath and in dressing are distressed at the way they behave when a nurse is employed. They often wonder why it is that children get so upset even to the point where they *can't bear the sight of that nurse's face.*

Grandfathers, too (and very often fathers), come in as carpenters in the building up of rages. Some grandfathers and now and then bachelor friends, too, are quite eager to have young children show them affection. If the child doesn't stop his play and run to his grandfather for a kiss, he *grasps the child as he passes and sometimes holds him against all struggles and forces him into an embrace or to sit on his lap.* If this happens a few times (I have watched many of these cases in the making) the child will begin to swerve aside four or five feet when he romps by his grandfather's chair. By so doing he keeps constantly out of reach. Then these adult murderers of a child's disposition say— "This child is frightfully rude. He has no natural affection. Your system of raising him is all wrong. How will the child ever learn to be affectionate?" Forcing a woman or a child into an affectionate embrace is pretty poor technique! It speedily defeats the very thing one wishes to encourage. The child so mistreated will continue to avoid that person and every one who speaks, looks or behaves like him. As he gets older he will avoid him by words when he has them at his command, by saying "Go away, I don't like you; I won't kiss you; I won't give you a hug," just as he avoids him when younger by keeping out of his reach.

Probably a good deal of this conditioning carries over into adult life. It is very probable that it is at the root of a lot of our first reactions to strangers. How often have you heard the expression, "I don't like that woman," "I don't like that man," "I just instinctively know that I could never get along with him or her." If we knew the genetic history of the speaker we could account for his so-called "instinctive" likes and dislikes of people. They are not instinctive. They are built in.

You can easily see how the home, day by day, complicates this side of the child's emotional life. It is constantly building in new rages and strengthening the old. Suppose we examine a few cases.

I am often called into conference over children who will not eat this or that—who dawdle over their food. Here is such a case: A beautiful little girl three years of age required the whole household to get her to eat. They asked me to take her in hand and to make recommendations. I first watched the eating performance through a crack in the door. The child was eating in her play room. She had eaten there all her life. This play room was a repository of at least five hundred toys. The nurse was old and fussy. She was the kind

who had raised seven of her own and, therefore, knew how to "raise" children. Here is
part of what I saw and heard. I can give you
only a little of the conversation.

"Dearie, here's your nice dinner—nice
cereal and milk. You are going to eat like a
nice girl tonight, aren't you?"

The child took a spoonful or two, then began to hold the spoon in mid air gazing in admiration at her pile of toys—then she day-
dreamed away for a time and next began a
soliloquy addressed to the empty air. The
nurse broke in and took the spoon out of her
hand roughly and began to shovel food down
her throat amid struggles, saying, "You are a
bad girl. Martha will go away and leave you
if you don't hurry up and eat your food."
Then followed a long line of "nice girls" with
forced feedings. Such had been her mealtimes
since the child first began to eat alone. Is it
any wonder that it took one hour to get her
to down a bowl of cereal, a small piece of
bread and a cup of milk? Is it any wonder

that the child slipped into day dreams to escape?

Something like this goes on in many homes. For this case I prescribed a change in the whole feeding régime. I asked the parents to discharge the old nurse and to get one who didn't know how to talk baby talk and one who had enough sense not to talk very much anyway while a child is performing a definite part of its daily routine. I asked them to let the child eat down in the dining room *alone*. I stipulated that if the child refused to accept this routine and went into a temper tantrum she was to be taken to her own room where she could cry herself out without an audience. Then when good temper was restored again, she was to be given one more trial at the food and if the same thing happened again, she had to go without that meal. I next stipulated that the mother should take a six weeks' vacation.

A complete and speedy cure resulted.

Naturally, you want to be sure when trying

out a procedure of this kind that nothing is organically wrong with your child before you use this method. Again, you do not want to make the child miss more than three meals in succession. Your physician should approve this course first, but be sure that you have a doctor for your child who is a real student of child behavior before you take his advice. The country is full of medical old fogies who will give you the kind of advice you are looking for rather than the kind you ought to have.

What are the sticking points in the day's routine?

In our recent work carried out at the Heckscher Foundation in New York Mrs. Mary Cover Jones observed a group of nine toddlers from seven in the morning when they woke up to seven at night when they went to bed. Without taking part in any of their activities, she followed them around all day,

day after day, noting carefully everything which brought on temper tantrums. We noted as rage or temper response any flare up or struggle that occurred in the absence of any physical hurt (that is, where no actual pain stimulus was present). We carried out this rather laborious and time-consuming test to see whether we could not locate some of the sticking points in the child's environment. Having located them, we hoped to be able to remove them, and if removal was not possible, to see if some modification of routine might not prove helpful. We hoped in this way to be able to get something of value for the home itself.

Here are the things that most frequently start the temper rows in children. They are listed in the order of their importance in the daily life of the child:

(1) Having to sit on the toilet chair

(2) Having property snatched away by some other child

(3) Having the face washed

(4) Working at something which won't pan out

(5) Being dressed

(6) Being undressed

(7) Being bathed

These nine toddlers varied in age from eighteen months to three years. During the day they all lived together. Many other situations called out temper fits, in all something like a hundred were noted. Any mother can add to this list from her own experience. There are few of us who have not had to give children medicine which they objected to. The administration of castor oil by the vise-like grip on hands, legs, feet, and even nose is familiar to all.

In making a study of this kind, you will find immediately that the child is always more difficult to handle if there are organic disturbances. Sleepy, hungry and colicky babies are always fit subjects for building in temper tantrums. Temper fits can be much more easily aroused in the child that has been shut in the house for days.

What can we do to keep down this flourishing crop of temper?

Obviously children must have a bath, must go to the toilet, must have their ears and noses cleaned out, even though temper tantrums do occur.

The first step is obvious. The child for the first year must be handled very gently. Some nurses and mothers develop a marvelous technique and deftness, a softness of touch. Yet they do not have to slight their work nor do they unduly linger over these operations. Nor do they buzz with infant chatter while handling the child. They never coddle it or shush it. Infant nurses in hospitals vary greatly in their ability to handle infants successfully. It is unfortunate that mothers have no opportunity to learn this technique in maternity wards. Some day we will have a real school for motherhood with a nursery attached where practical experience can be had in handling infants and children under the instruction of a nurse who has developed a satisfactory technique.

Next, we have yet to learn much regarding the kind of clothing children should wear during the infancy period. I have paid my respects to modern ways of dressing children at the beginning of this chapter. I lay no claim to being an expert in infants' layettes. I merely want to register certain psychological objections to some of the articles of infant wear now in common use. It seems to me that if mothers were willing to forego lingerie dresses and white petticoats and sweaters and long stockings during the early months of infancy and would be content to dress the baby in looser clothes, the dressing and undressing of children would be a more tranquil operation than at present. They would be equally comfortable during the day and the garments could be made so as to yield adequate warmth.

Then, too, cannot the usual diaper band and shirt be combined into one garment with loose sleeves, made like a shirt buttoning down the front with two heavy tabs reënforced for tying or pinning the diaper to on each side? Then, following the best hospital practice but not yet in general use in the home, the diaper should be put on square and tied on each side. This gives the infant more space for movement. Cannot we get along with one flannel petticoat made loose and sleeveless with two buttons buttoning down the front? Cannot we follow this with a muslin slip made equally loose with kimona sleeves instead of the usual dainty tightfitting ones? This should have no more than two buttons and should button in front. And is there any reason why young babies should wear socks or stockings before they begin to walk? There are two children under my observation who were brought up to an age where they could stand alone (9 to 10 months) without shoes or socks —and to the sitting up age (6 to 7 months) without sweaters—and neither of these children ever had a cold during the first six months of their lives.

The most practical advice one can give the nurse or mother is to *let the child learn as quickly as possible to do everything for itself*. The child can learn to feed itself at quite an early age, the average child at about eighteen months. In a month to six weeks time thereafter it should become fairly proficient in getting all of its food to its mouth with a spoon. At twenty to twenty-two months you can begin to replace the spoon with a blunt fork. A bottle fed baby can easily be weaned at from six to eight months. It can be taught to drink directly from a cup. It should begin to drink without assistance about the eighteenth month. Hunger will do wonders; patience for a few days or weeks will do the rest. The child should begin to sit on a regular toilet fitted with folded child's seat with no one in the room with it from about nine months of age on. Children should begin to bathe themselves with the nurse nearby at three years of age. Naturally for weeks and months the mother and nurse will have to take a hand in finishing the job on eyes, ears, nose and back. It is surprising how quickly a child can learn to clean out its nose—even efficiently and safely but naturally always under the mother's eyes. The child can begin to blow its nose from about the twentieth month on—to blow when you say "blow." Blowing the nose, however, is a slow growth in most children. They should be pretty efficient in brushing their teeth at twenty-one months.

The child should begin to dress itself at 2½ years of age. One has to start very slowly and be very patient. For example, a child at twenty months can put on its bed room slippers. It can put on its stockings with some expert assistance at even two years of age. At three years of age the child can step into its underwear and put its arms through and step into its trousers. At that age it cannot do much with buttons unless given a great amount of special practice. (Why buttons should ever have been placed in the exact center of the back on any child's dress is more than a psychologist can explain). Even at 3 years he still needs a little help putting on his stockings. He should be able at 3 to put on his shoes. At 3½ he can get on his outer clothes or any sweater that does not pull on over his head. He can, however, take off the latter type of sweater. While not very proficient in buttoning, he can unfasten buttons that have reasonably loose buttonholes. At 3 years, the boy should be able to stand up at the toilet to micturate. If supplied with flashlight and chamber, he should be able to get up during the night for this purpose, practically never wetting the bed thereafter or disturbing the sleep of nurse and parents. At 3½ years of age, any child whose clothes are first unfastened should be able without assistance to mount and sit down upon the toilet seat of adults.

At four years of age even a boy should be

able completely to dress himself—given time and no hurrying. The one exception I would make here is tying his shoes. That seems to offer considerable difficulty. He should be able thoroughly to brush his teeth, to gargle, to use an eye cup when necessary, brush his own hair, put on his greatcoat and his gloves— he cannot do much with boots and rubbers. He can use knife and fork and butter his own bread—I have seen this latter operation done fairly well at 3 years. In general at this age children should begin to dress and act like youthful men and women and should be scrupulously treated as such.

The problem of dressing and undressing during this period would be much more easily solved if some skilled behaviorist with a penchant for becoming a couturier for infants should experiment on making clothes which toddlers themselves can operate. But even with all our care in dressing and in handling, infants and young children will occasionally develop temper tantrums. There are too many things not under the control even of the careful parent which make for it.

Is there any experimental way to *uncondition* them, to remove a temper the way we can remove a fear? We have not yet had the opportunity to make this study. There are certain indications that such a method can be devised, but until it has been tried out and found to work, there is not much use in giving way to speculation.

CHAPTER FIVE

NIGHT AND DAYTIME CARE OF THE CHILD

UNTIL the child is two he belongs to the home. At two he goes out under his own power to see the world. To get along in this new world he must enter it prepared.

How shall we get him ready? He is not born ready. He has absolutely no instincts of cleanliness. Indeed many infra-human animals would hesitate to associate with him. And yet "polite" society demands "nice" habits, conventions and customs. He must start with cleanly personal habits—must keep his face and hands washed and his clothes clean. He must put on certain eating habits with knife, fork and spoon. To say "Yes, thank you, Mrs. Jones," "I am sorry, Mrs. Smith, but my mother asked me not to." To keep his temper when teased—not to snatch toys from playmates—not to bolt his food—not to talk all the time. To be "brave" but not foolhardy—never to "strike a woman." And to do and not to do all the millions of things a gentleman or a lady should do or not do.

The number of reactions that have to be built in and kept in seems endless. But we should not despair. The time was when we used to think it took generations to make a well-bred person. Now we know parents can do it in a few months' time if they start to cultivate the garden before the weeds begin to grow.

While no one can lay down a hard and fast routine of infant and child care which will fit every home, still certain general plans can be made and adhered to. Here are some suggestions for the 2–5 year old child.

Routine of Night and Daytime Care

The Bath: Unless counseled otherwise by your physician 7 P. M. is a good bedtime for the ages 2–5 years. Before bed comes a tepid bath at 5:30 P. M. The bath should be a se-

rious but not gloomy occasion. The object of
the bath is to get the child clean and not to en-
tertain it. Many mothers fill the tub full of
celluloid toys and prolong the bath to a degree which is useless and foolish. The child
cries when he has to get out—gets so interested
in his water games that he never heeds your
instructions in the art of washing and caring
for himself. He should be taught as early as
a year old to use a wash cloth on himself and
at 3½ years of age he should be able to do
most of the job alone. Of course, from the beginning he must be handled gently and quietly
otherwise a slight accident such as slipping
under water may condition him against his
bath for a long time. The water in the tub
should be not more than 4 to 8 inches deep
depending upon the age of the child, and he
should never be left in it alone until he has
reached the age of six years at least.

But don't make the bath a nightmare by
rough handling and carelessness. In cleaning
the young one's ears for instance one needs

all kinds of ingenuity and patience; in washing his hair, a little soap in his eyes may create a permanent emotional disturbance at having his hair washed. Great care must be taken in washing the sex organs—although they must be thoroughly and gently cleaned—any continued handling of them may start masturbation on the child's part. Boys who have not been circumcised should be taught to push back the foreskin about three times a week and wash the underlying tissues thoroughly. They can start to do this at the age of 3½ to 4 years.

Two children should never be bathed in the same tub—whether they are of the same or different sexes—although there should be no inhibitions about their seeing each other naked in or out of the bath.

After the bath the child should be thoroughly dried with a soft bath towel. When he is young it is best to pat him dry. When his body gets toughened gentle rubbing of the back, legs and arms is advisable.

After drying, many hospitals and pediatricians advocate for children under 2 months of age the use of a first grade olive oil or mineral oil with no powder. After two months, powder may be used but with caution—always keeping the baby's head turned away from the powder box, lest his nasal passages be irritated and he sneeze. If the creases and buttocks are irritated at all they should be treated with olive oil by putting a few drops on a piece of absorbent cotton and rubbing the surface gently. The parts so treated are not powdered but only the rest of the body—the powder being lightly sprinkled on and gently rubbed. The child should never be allowed to play with a powder box full or empty. It is a bad habit to establish.

Some hospitals advocate for the infant's skin neither oil nor powder but only warm water, castile soap and thorough drying. The skin of some children is sensitive to olive oil. In this case your physician should be consulted.

After the bath comes a light meal of your physician's choosing.

Before bedtime play

Then comes a half hour of quiet play. In many homes where more than one child is present, before bedtime is group romping time. This I believe is wrong—it is poor preparation for quiet sleeping. I find that children when allowed to romp are loath to leave exciting play. They whine and bad discipline results. Sleep is delayed which leads to the children singing, talking to themselves, getting up and running about and calling out to each other. The child, who after supper plays quietly with pencil, paper, crayons, clay, or is read to, goes to bed with little protest and drops into a restful sleep much more quickly. This is a good time to give the father his half hour. It keeps the children used to male society. Then, too, they have their chance to ply him with questions.

Should children take toys to bed?

Should the children be allowed to take anything to bed with them? ask many mothers.
It is a sloppy habit and one easy to get into
yet very hard to break.

Of course, no serious harm is done the child
if it is allowed to go to bed with one or two
toys. Indeed there is one argument often urged
in its favor. If the child doesn't go to sleep at
once it has something to play with—and since
it wakes up in the morning before it is allowed
to get up, it again has something to play with.
It is, therefore, less tempted to explore its own
body. But it often happens when this is allowed that the habit is carried on long beyond
the time when such infant behavior should be
abandoned. Often such habits are carried over
into adult life. Then they may become trou-
blesome.

The final look before turning out the light

Every mother should give faithful atten-

tion to bedtime régime. Before leaving the
room see that everything you customarily allow the child is at hand—that he has had his
drink of water—that he was placed upon the
toilet—that his chamber is under his bed and
that his flashlight for getting up at night is
under his pillow. His bed should be low
enough for him to get in and out of easily
from the time he is 2 years old. Take a
last look at his clothes to see that everything
is in order—that he is not too warm—that
his hands are placed outside the cover (if he
is not a thumb sucker, inside if he is)—then
a pat on the head, a quiet good night—lights
out and door closed. If he howls, let him howl.
A week of this régime will give you an orderly bedtime.

If it can possibly be avoided never let children sleep together in the same room. Each
child should have a separate room. No nurse
or other adult should ever sleep in the same
room with infant or child. Unless these conditions can be met no woman should be blamed

in my opinion if she refuses to consent to have a child.

Waking up time

Morning and bedlam?—No. Modern training calls always for an orderly life. Usually from 1 year of age to 3 pediatricians specify that orange juice shall be given when the child wakes up in the morning. Children who sleep properly awaken on a schedule. The waking time can easily be set for 6: 30. The orange juice should then be given regularly at that hour every morning, the child put on the toilet for the relief of the bladder (only). Put the child back to bed and allow it to sit up in bed and play quietly alone with one or two chosen toys. It should be taken up at 7 o'clock, sponged lightly, dressed and given its breakfast at 7: 30; then allowed to romp until 8, then put upon the toilet for 20 minutes or less (until the bowel movement is complete). The infant from 8 months of age onward should have a special toilet seat into which he can be safely strapped. *The child should be left in the bathroom without toys and with the door closed.* Under no circumstances should the door be left open or the mother or nurse stay with the child. This is a rule which seems to be almost universally broken. When broken it leads to dawdling, loud conversation, in general to unsocial and dependent behavior.

Early morning activities

As soon as possible in the morning the child should be put into a sunny room (some day every home will have a nursery fitted with a skylight which will admit the ultra-violet rays so that sun-baths can be taken naked even in the dead of winter) to play until the mother or nurse has done her household duties. He should be taught to stay there and play or work quietly alone. On clear days he should be out of doors by ten o'clock. Where he goes and what he should do depend on the family situation. The important thing is that he should get systematic exercise. A good brisk walk with the nurse is excellent. Where there is no nurse and the mother has other duties he should have one toy such as a kiddie car, wagon, scooter, tricycle or skates, depending upon the age. He should exercise up and down the sidewalk in front of the house or in the back yard.

Of course changes in seasons bring changes in occupation. In winter the sled or ice skates must replace the bicycle. One very bad situation is developing among mothers who have automobiles. There is a tendency to let the child give up walking and exercising. The mother takes the child with her wherever she goes. Such a life makes the child little better than a helpless parasite. He gets no sunshine, he breathes gasoline fumes. He quarrels if he ever has to walk. His muscles have no chance to acquire skill.

Lunch and the nap afterwards

Luncheon or preferably dinner (midday) should be served to the child and nurse in the dining room. From 2 years on the child should be at ease with a fork and spoon so that he needs very little help and should get into the habit of eating at table and respecting adult habits. All such things as use of his napkin, hands in his lap, waiting for table to be cleared until dessert arrives, moderate low-pitched conversation, should begin to be inculcated at this age. If there is no nurse, the child should eat by himself. It isn't fair for the child to have to watch adults eat all kinds of food which he is not allowed to taste.

After lunch every child up to the age of 5 should have at least an hour's nap. Every child over 5 should have an hour for rest if not for sleep with perhaps one toy or a picture book if he can't sleep. Many parents when the children are very young and not very strong let them have the nap in the morning, from 11:00 to 12:30, and then have lunch. This routine sometimes considerably relieves quarrelsomeness, temper tantrums and the like.

Afternoon play and social contact

After the nap the child should go out again. *Social contacts* should have their place as part of the afternoon schedule: Games with other children on the street, in the park or in the home. Some systematic instruction should be given if the child cannot go to school before public school life begins. There is no reason why children as young as 3 to 4 shouldn't have instructions in boxing, baseball, football, tennis, dancing and nature study. Of course all this can be carried to extremes. The child's life must not be made into a series of engagements with no chance for uncensored play. Every home that has a right to house a child should have a back yard or be situated near a park where at least an hour of the day can be spent in play with companions. They should be let alone—fights, accidents, quarrels and all. For this period one should provide a tent, sand-pile, see-saw, swing, clay, and other simple objects. This spot should be **the** refuge of the child unvisited by the adult. In the spring and summer ask your physician to instruct you how to get him ready to have at least a half hour in the sunshine naked with his brothers and sisters or alone.

You may say that such a routine as is suggested here is impossible for the mother who has no nurse. This does not square with the facts. I have recently made a study of child routine in 20 homes. In two of those homes where infant care and routine were most perfect *there was neither a nurse nor any other servant.* It was most interesting to note in many of these homes that the routine put down in writing by the mother was almost never adhered to in practice and that even in homes of wealth where there was a nurse and other servants each mother was kind of an opportunist on routine. The lack of an intelligent plan consistently carried out was most appalling! I found children put to bed with bread in the crib so that when they woke up they would not cry; children put to bed in pairs until they fell asleep and then were separated; children allowed to eat at all hours; children of four whose mothers left them wet for hours, and had made no effort to train them even during waking hours; children of four and under who had to have some-one sit by until they fell asleep, whose mothers had to go to them six and seven times a night (perfectly well children at that) to quiet them and get them to sleep again.

Day and night time cleanliness

The establishment of even a well ordered day and night time routine does not solve all your problems. The problem of cleanliness should intrude itself almost from birth.

The teaching of continence in children is admittedly difficult. No one likes to see wet children and yet that seems to be their chronic state. Such incontinent acts in children are soon detected by older children on the outside. Incontinent children are laughed at, ridiculed and made scapegoats. Habits of inferiority and shyness are bred in and these results persist long after habits of continence are bred in. Even adults shun such children. The child gets his frowns and hard looks and even slaps long after the act is committed. This does no good. It is not possible to establish a conditioned response where the "shock" or punishment occurs so long after the response.

Before asking how such unsocial habits can be corrected we might ask, is there no way in *which we can keep them from forming?* It is quite easy to start habits of day time continence (conditioned responses) when the child is from 3–5 weeks old by putting the chamber to the child (*but at this age never on it*) each time it is aroused for feeding. It is often surprising how quickly the conditioned response is established if your routine is unremitting and your patience holds out.

Good practice differs as to whether you

should wake your child after 10 P. M. to place him upon a chamber. I believe very thoroughly in it but I do not believe in assisting the child very much. A good many mothers pick the child up (any age from 2–6), place the chamber under him, then put him back to bed and cover him up. The child often goes through the whole act without *ever waking* up. The plan of waking him gently but thoroughly by calling to him—telling him to get up—letting him go through everything unassisted, even to covering himself up again, works out very well. If this procedure is gone through quietly and gently it never disturbs sleep but for a moment. The child is usually asleep again before you can close the door. Gradually as the child gets older you can wake him slightly later each night until he can go through the whole night comfortably. The mother who neglects her child in the day time need not try to establish night time continence.

The other plan is to train the child to go

through the night from 7:30 P.M. to 7:30
A.M. Several children I have worked with
up to the age of 5 have gone through the night
since they were 2 years of age with rarely an
accident. In these children day time continence was perfected within the first 15
months.

Neglect by mother or nurse is usually the
cause of incontinence; the mother is too busy
to watch over it; she engages in half hour
telephone conversations; she visits and leaves
the children to the cook or to shift for themselves. The nurse gets too interested in talking
to other nurses to watch over her own charges.
Somehow nothing seems to make us take this
problem very seriously. We demand cleanliness in our cats and dogs from infancy yet
feel no shame when our 2 and 3 year old children go wet around the house and even out
in the street to join their playmates.

Sometimes, however, whether through neglect or through accident, habits of continence
do break down. If they are hard to reëstab-

lish, consult your child specialist: there are several bodily conditions which might cause it. When he has straightened these out—the habits may reassert themselves without reconditioning. Very likely not, however; if the child is below 5 or 6 years of age, retraining must be resorted to.

What to do when the habits break down? We have much to learn about reëstablishing habits of continence.

Here is the case of a boy aged 4—continent day and night with rare night accidents since the age of 2. He goes on a two weeks' visit to his grandparents where the oversight is not unremitting. This child had always been taken up at 10–11 o'clock each night. The habit broke down. After his return to his home, bed-wetting became pernicious. Even if taken up two or three times at night he would be wet in the morning. The mother and father tried "reasoning," and "nice boy" arguments—unavailingly. Then social banishment was next tried. The father and mother refused to talk to the child during the day if the bed had been wet during the night. Next severe scoldings were indulged in by the parents—first by the mother alone and then by the father. Then came punishment—spanking upon the buttocks. These methods were totally unavailing. Next they made the child wash out its own pajamas each day. This soon became a joke and even his 2½ year old brother laughed with him as they started for the tub. When the case was brought to me I asked the parents and nurse absolutely to ignore the accidents—to say nothing at any time, morning, noon or night. But to reward him each morning if no accident occurred. The child was inordinately fond of chewing gum, so he was given one piece each no-accident day. Under no other circumstances could he get even so much as a taste of chewing gum (candy was never allowed). Improvement occurred almost immediately but nearly two months elapsed before the habit of continence was completely restored. This case is typical of many. In all that I have worked on a reward has proven most effective. It works its cure rather slowly, however. We still have much to learn about the handling of this problem.

Thumb sucking

In the process of socializing your child another problem often comes up. It is thumb sucking or hand or finger sucking. This highly unsocial act is difficult to control if it gets a good start in early infancy. Sometimes an object is sucked such as a piece of cloth, an old blanket or other covers. When the mother is very careless the nipple of the nursing bottle is persistently sucked and later chewed after the milk has been consumed. Millions of mothers who are almost criminally careless use a pacifier to keep the child quiet. The child sucks it all during his waking hours.

There is nothing to be alarmed about in early thumb sucking. Many infants are born almost with a finger in the mouth. This is due to their position *in utero*. If you will watch the new born youngsters for a few months after birth you will see the result of this pre-birth position of the hands. Rarely does the infant move the hands below the waist line. Hence it is natural that the mouth should be "discovered" before any other part of the body. He discovers it by the usual "trial and error" method. Trial movements cease when the fingers touch the mouth. Then sucking movements immediately begin. Sucking movements do not have to be learned. They are well established in most infants at birth (or shortly thereafter). *In other words, thumb sucking is a now familiar conditioned response connected with eating.* The lips belong to the general area of the sex field too, so that in part thumb sucking is a sex response (using this word in its broad modern sense) closely akin to masturbation which is a habit even infants may form.

If persistent thumb sucking is in part a

food habit, we should expect to find it most persisted in by children who are continually hungry or whose bodies are not kept free from irritation. You will see this view supported in every poorly run orphan or nursery home.

Why should we fight against it? In the first place, it reflects upon the training and care the parent gives the child. Parents whose children suck their thumbs are condemned in progressive communities.

From the standpoint of the child the matter is serious. Physicians tell us that some 90% of disease due to germs find their way into the body through the mouth. The child with its mobile hands gathers germs everywhere. Next it puts the hands into the warm, moist mouth. The germs are thus given an ideal breeding place.

If persisted in for long at any early age before the bony, tendinous and muscular tissues harden, the mouth becomes misshapen and the fingers and hands are changed in their contours. There are many other bodily changes which may occur, such as interference with the proper growth and position of the teeth.

The effect of thumb sucking upon the child's personality is the most serious aspect of all. It is an infantile type of reaction which when carried over beyond the age of infancy ends in a pernicious habit almost impossible to break. Indeed if carried through adolesence in the modified form of nail biting, finger biting, cuticle picking or finger picking, it becomes practically impossible to break. It is then classed as a neurotic trait.

The act brings with it a kind of soothing or quieting effect like a drug. As long as the individual is allowed to engage in it he is perfectly docile in all of his reactions. Scold him about it, try to check it and he becomes irritable and uneasy. Apparently when the child has his fingers in his mouth *he is,* speaking broadly, *blocked to all other stimuli.* Hence the persistent thumb sucker cannot be as easily made to respond to toys and other objects upon which we normally train children. The outside world doesn't get a good chance at him. He doesn't conquer his world. He becomes an "exclusive," an auto-erotic. With his fingers safely in his mouth the child may sometimes not even react to dangerous stimuli. Our own experiments at Johns Hopkins show that even when stimuli which are known to produce fright are shown to the thumb sucking child they lose their power to arouse him.

How can we correct thumb sucking? The answer is, *cure it during the first few days of infancy.* Watch the baby carefully the first few days. Keep the hands away from the mouth as often as you are near the baby in its waking moments. And always when you put it into its crib for sleep, see that the hands are tucked inside the covers—and if you examine the sleeping infant from time to time see when you leave it that the hands are under the covers (when the child gets older—over one year of age—you will want to see that the hands are left *outside* the covers when put to bed the reason for which will appear on page 175).

If the habit develops in spite of this early scrutiny, consult your physician about the infant's diet. Tell him about the thumb sucking. If after changes in the diet thumb sucking persists, then take more drastic steps to break the habit. Sew loose white, canton flannel mitts with no finger or thumb divisions to the sleeves of the night gown and on all the *day dresses, and leave them on for two weeks or more—day and night.* So many mothers leave them on only at night. Unless the child is watched every moment the hand will at one time or another get back to the mouth. You must be careful to see that the dress or night gown is fastened securely but not tightly at the throat—else if the infant is persistent he will learn to disrobe himself to get at his hands. If the habit still persists make the material of the mitts of rougher and rougher material.

I have tried many methods that will not work. Those clumsy aluminum mitts are ineffective. The child bangs himself over the head and eyes and nine times out of ten gets out of them in one way or another. Pasteboard tubes over the elbow joint are used in some good hospitals but they are cruel. The child cannot rub an irritation or scare away a fly or mosquito. Coating the fingers with bitter aloes has never worked out for me. Occasionally the infant goes right ahead without baulking at the aloes, or if he does make a wry face or two he soon goes on serenely. I've never had any success with taping the finger. Either he picks the tape off after a time (if one year of age or over) or else sucks the finger, tape and all.

I have tried punishment—sharply rapping the finger with a pencil. This is beautifully effective while the experimenter is around but at night the habit reasserts itself. Scolding and corporal punishment likewise have proved wholly ineffective.

Destructiveness

Still another problem we meet in socializing our children is that of *destructiveness;* dishes, vases, lamps, bric-a-brac—nothing is sacred or safe. It is brought about largely by our allowing them to misuse their toys. During the course of childhood nearly every child breaks up hundreds of dollars' worth of toys. In one family consisting of two boys, one 5 the other 3, I took a rough record of the amount of money spent in toys during five years. Approximately $800 had been spent by family and friends. A rough inventory showed that the few toys remaining at the end of the fifth year did not have a value of over $25. But the economic waste is not the important feature. The toys were so poorly made and chosen so poorly with respect to the children's ages that *destructive toy habits* were formed. The children no sooner saw them than they began their work of destruction. I visit, usually, several families with children on Xmas day and note the number of slaughtered toys. It is not a foolish guess to say that many millions of dollars' worth of property are destroyed each Xmas day. Destroyed as utterly as were high explosives in the World War. And with just as poor results socially. Children should be taught conservation and use of property as early in life as they begin to possess property. Naturally children take objects apart to examine their workings but this requires some technical skill and the child that takes a toy apart to examine it should be taught just as carefully to put it together again. Think of children of one and two or even three years given watches—even of the dollar kind. Think of their being given expensive electric trains— and expensive and delicate models of airplanes and motor boats and phonographs— all worth while toys for the boy and girl who is old enough to handle them—but marked for 24 hour slaughter when given to children too young.

Too many toys

Neatness and order must be instilled early if it is ever to be instilled. Children with toys all over the floor do not have time at the end of the day to clear them all up carefully—handle them gently and stack them away in order. You buy a toy box but the toys are dumped in by the armful and thrown about the room at random the next day until the child comes upon the one he wants.

Again nearly all the toys are made to be run only by an adult. I tried the other day to buy a top which a 3 year old could wind and release. Only after much effort did I discover it. A test in the shops show hundreds of trains with springs so short that they will run only after an adult with effort winds them. Dumping wagons and carts galore are found that only the adult can work, airplanes and motor boats that mother has to call father in to operate. Here again we teach the child dependence.

There are several very definite things we can do about it.

(1) Don't let the children have too many toys at a time. If too many are sent either send them back or distribute them to less fortunate families or put them away without letting the children see them. Let them wring every bit of organization and amusement they can get out of what they do have before giving them others. And curtail still more if the few they have are not well handled, used, and cleared away at night.

(2) Choose the toy for the age. Study the child for this. Children vary so in their manual skill. Many children under one year like nothing better than small boxes they can open and close—preferably metal and wooden boxes which have been used for something in the household. They like cloth dolls and animals. They are considerably shaped during this first year (during all years of course) by the activity patterns of the family. What children "like" to play with is largely due to this

and to the way they are handled and by the patterns set by playmates.

(3) Choose only well made toys. You can't control the kinds of toys your friends send your children but you can decide whether the child is to have them. There are hundreds of well made toys now. Blocks—of stone and wood. Metal toys for building. Every year the profusion of toys is greater. If you buy only substantial toys, manufacturers will soon learn to build them better. In studying the toy problem I have examined several hundred toys. Among them are many where parts are held together with bolts and nuts. Never once have I found a wagon, for example, where the manufacturer took the trouble to bruise the thread on the bolt a bit after the nut was tightened to keep the nut from gradually loosening, or to enlarge the head of the bolt to keep the nut from falling off if the nut should by accident become loosened. One tap of the hammer with a sharp instrument held against the thread after the nut is screwed up

will keep it on for always. As a consequence
of this carelessness every vacant lot contains
remains of toy wagons, bicycles and carts.
The nuts came off, the toy broke down and
soon was discarded.

Teach the child to make his own toys

Feeding the child only on ready made toys
tends to break down his own efforts to construct objects. Every behaviorist loves to see
the child begin to construct objects from raw
material. Encouragement—*dearth of ready
made toys* and *being surrounded* by raw material, such as *wood, clay, nails, screws,* and
two or three simple instruments, such as hammer and saw and later a plane are the essen-
tials needed to stimulate the child to make
his own playthings. What wonderful artistry
in woodworking has been accomplished with
a chisel and wooden mallet! What wonderful
draughting with a rule, a pen, pencil and pair
of dividers! What wonderful paintings with
a brush and a few tubes of paint!

An easy first step to lead the child into using raw materials is the toy which comes in knock down form and can readily be put together by children as young as 4 years of age. Many excellent unpainted wooden toys of this kind can now be had in wagons, automobiles and the like.

What I am heading for is the building in of habits of ingenuity, of skill and craftsmanship—a fostering of the apprenticeship spirit early (now so nearly gone even in the life of our adults).

But since we should give the child some toys let us see to it that they are well made, suited to his age and that he *wants them* enough to use them properly and carefully. There are several schools now where considerable attention is given to this. But I know of no homes even trying to solve the problem. In a few schools the child is shown a case containing a large number of toys suited to his age and skill. He is allowed to select one and only one. He plays with that toy alone during his play period and *no other*. And when the play period is over he has to put it away. This system is worthy of adoption in every home.

Inculcating a respect for toys almost always does away with the problem of destructiveness.

The problem of getting and keeping a nurse

But will our nurses carry out our plans? Many busy mothers tell me that all plans for child training, however sensible, are useless because nurses will not carry them out. Nurses are the weakest link in infant culture today. They are untrained, green and poorly mannered. They are either bullies or sentimentalists. It is no unusual thing for a home to have a succession of five nurses per year—nor for a child to have had from 25–40 nurses and governesses from birth to 12 years of age. If the nurses were good the fact that the child had been in the hands of forty of them would not be detrimental—possibly quite otherwise because it would tend to keep down fixations.

There seems to be nothing to do but train our nurses after we get them into the home. Many of them resent this—if they have ever had another job, they think they know how to "manage" children. A mother taking a new nurse will save time and energy in the end by working with the nurse daily and hourly for two weeks. This will tend to weaken the nurse's hold but when you find that she is reasonably well-trained you should leave the children to her care until her control has been reestablished.

The main consideration after the nurse has taken charge is that there be no divided authority. "Mother says I can do it." "Mother always lets me do it." Then the call to the mother— "Mother can't I do it—nurse says I can't." No self respecting nurse can stay long in such a home.

The problem of getting and keeping a good nurse will remain unsolvable until better material can be induced to go in for nursing and until we have behavioristic schools for nurses. Six months' training in the actual handling of children from 2–6 under the eye of competent instructors should make a fairly satisfactory child's nurse. To keep them we should let the position of nurse or governess in the home be a respected one. Where the mother herself must be the nurse—which is the case in the vast majority of American homes —she must look upon herself while performing the functions of a nurse as a professional woman and not as a sentimentalist masquerading under the name of "Mother."

Is the end result worth the struggle?

Is it worth all this struggle—won't the child get along anyway—haven't millions got along before busy-bodies stepped in to tell us how to rear our youngsters? If all of these things have to be done doesn't it mean that motherhood is becoming almost a profession? I believe the struggle is worth while even if the mother does have to turn professional.

The end result is a *happy child free as air* because he has mastered the stupidly simple
demands society makes upon him. *An independent* child because all during his training
you have made him play and work alone a
part of the time, and you have made him get
out of difficulties by his own efforts. *A child
that meets and plays with other children*
frankly, openly, untroubled by shyness and inferiority. *An original child* because his perfect adjustment to his environment gives him
leisure to experiment. Don't believe anyone
who tells you that such insistence on routine
tends to steam roller the child and to reduce
the growth of his own "inward life and
powers." "Spontaneity," "inward development," and the like are phrases used by those
too lazy or too stupid or too prejudiced to
study children in the actual making.

The only person in life who is effectively
original is the person who has a routine and
has mastered a technique. The person who

has not these is a slave—his life is taken up in trying to keep up with the procession of those struggling to obtain just bread, meat, and a roof for shelter.

CHAPTER SIX

WHAT SHALL I TELL MY CHILD ABOUT
SEX?

WHY is it so difficult for parents to tell their children about sex?

One reason is that many parents realize that their own knowledge of sex is so inadequate and so unscientific that they doubt their right to talk to their children.

There is yet a deeper reason. Most of us have secured our knowledge about sex in a round-about, hazy way—from older children, from none too scrupulous nurses and from sentimental parents who talked in metaphors. We get confused when we try to talk to our children. Common sense deserts us. We put the children off when they question us and say, "Some day when you are older you can understand, then I'll tell you all about it."

The result is that our children get their

"knowledge" in the same round-about way we did. They put on the same secretive attitude we put on in our youth. They are told by older playmates that they must never tell their parents what they have learned on the street and in back yards. When parents cannot put off the conventional talk they think they ought to have with their children, they try to get the child to listen. But the child by this time is diffident. She tries to avoid the subject. She gets confused—will not answer questions. She has heard many garbled versions and she has become secretive. The parent construes this as a good sign. "My poor innocent lamb is ignorant about sex—I could hardly get her to listen to me. Isn't it sweet that she is so unspoiled and so pure?"

Their innocent lambs have been learning about sex (using the term broadly) from the time their wavering footsteps at two years took them into groups of four and six year old children. But the ban of silence has been put upon their lips by older children. The book is closed to a parent who has too long neglected them. Just because your child will not talk to you gives you little reason for believing that sex is not a topic of conversation with its playmates.

Here is a word for word conversation I overheard today between a boy aged 5 and a girl aged 7.

"Grace, will you marry me?"

"I don't know Sammie, I am too old for you."

"But Grace if you will marry me I will build you a house at Long Beach and I'll buy you an automobile with red wheels."

"Thank you, Sammie, but I want to choose my own automobile. I guess I will marry you though."

Sammie was overjoyed. "And Sammie, we will have children, won't we?"

"You will, Grace. I won't have any. Men don't have children. But how will we get them, Grace?"

"I don't know, Sammie."

Such a conversation does not show that these two children were precocious or unduly curious about sex. They are here trying to piece together their chance facts into a kind of philosophy of life. One of the first problems in this scheme is where do children come from.

What would have been easier than to have taken these two bright children at this point and talked to them about the origin of children?

I asked the mother of the 7 year old girl why she hadn't told her daughter more about sex. Her answer was that she had neither the knowledge nor the courage.

Where can the mother, who is inadequately prepared, find enlightenment? Unfortunately the knowledge is difficult to obtain. There are few books which can be trusted. There are few medical men who have adequate knowledge of sex, fewer still who have that detailed objectivity of thought so necessary in imparting information. It is a world beset by super-

stition—filled with old wives' tales that will
not down—loaded with sentiment and reli-
gion. To understand the subject thoroughly
one must know the simple facts about the psychopathology of everyday life. I once wrote
to eighty distinguished physicians and asked
them point blank whether the average physician (medical practitioner) could be de-
pended upon to give sane instruction to our
young people. The answer in most cases was
"no." I quote, without mentioning their names,
from three of our distinguished physicians:

Dr. A—— "No. The average medical practitioner never heard the word sex men-
tioned in medical school and has never
discussed any sex problems with anyone.
He is himself shocked at mention of the
subject. He is not tolerant of a sex emo-
tion as such, but he tolerates the idea of
venereal disease."

Dr. B—— "My experience is that he is a

great prude and knows little of the psychology of sex. He has a narrow orthodoxy which is mostly false."

Dr. C—— "I do not believe the average medical practitioner is any more competent to give sex instruction to children than are the average parents."

The data gathered from this study form a real indictment against the general mass of medical men. They show the real superstition and ignorance about one of the fundamental problems of life on the part of men we have been taught to revere.

On the other hand this same study revealed that most of the psychopathologists (the medically trained psychoanalysts and the psychiatrists) had a thoroughly sane, wholesome and adequate point of view. My advice to any father or mother with children is to go to the psychopathologist for one, two, or more hours of instruction, if you feel that your own knowledge is inadequate. If you have the slightest embarrassment when you talk to your children—if you are ever angered or embarrassed by what your children may do or say to you or to others, then your knowledge is insufficient and you should supplement it.

Let us consider just one fact here which proves almost conclusively that 75% of the mothers (and naturally an equal number of fathers) are not competent to guide their children without some outside help. It is well known that possibly not more than 25 percent. of the married women have sufficient knowledge of sex and training in sex to experience the full value of the sex relationship. Physiologically these women are normal but their mother's training makes them inadequate. This means that only one mother in four really understands sex well enough to talk to her child about it. It means that three out of four go on giving their sons and daughters a dwarfed, starved and generally inadequate picture of the husband and wife relationship.

A vicious cycle has been established and a whirlwind of divorce, neurasthenia, melancholia and invalidism is reaped.

So before taking your children in hand see that your knowledge is full—accurate, objective and free from sentiment of every kind. If it has not this characteristic and you have not the courage to make it adequate and objective, then by all means get someone else to instruct your child. Mothers and fathers, however, are the logical ones to instruct their children. The child has a right to expect the parents to do it if he is to continue to give them his homage and respect. Their failure to prepare themselves to impart this knowledge is one of the greatest problems we have today in social hygiene. During the past few years remarkable progress has been made in the education of parents. Probably a generation or two will be needed to complete the work. The greatest handicap to the work is the fact that due to prudery our great newspapers and magazines are afraid to print the needed instructions. Until lately it has been possible to reach the public only through books and leaflets and lectures in medical clinics. The spread of information is consequently slow.

Almost any mother if she starts when her child is young enough and wholeheartedly undertakes this problem can gradually acquire a good objective technique. She should form the habit when her child is *two* years of age of talking things out. Two or three times a week she should set aside a half hour period to get acquainted with the way her child's life is being organized—not just along sex lines but along every line. She should, as it were, take an inventory from time to time of the child's verbal consolidations. She should invite questions about the child's universe and patiently answer his whys—what makes the clock go—why does the watch tick—where does the sun go at night? What makes the thunder? From two to five the child is a living question mark. This is the mother and father's golden opportunity to establish *rapport.*

If these whys are answered sensibly, the child begins to believe that parents are reliable sources of information. Older children from less careful families are only too eager to try out their hand at instructing younger children. They make it interesting too. Parental information must be able to compete in interest with this "under cover" information or else your hold is gone. Interest in this type of information shows up even in the adult. A few years ago our great dailies gave us all needed information about scandal, divorce and murder cases. Recently tabloid newspapers made under cover gossip articulate. The world jumped at it. A startling growth in circulation has taken place surpassing anything ever known before to newspaperdom. The analogy does not need to be drawn any closer. If the parent is to compete with the outside he must make his information *interesting*.

You may feel that since you are sending your child to kindergarten all of its questions should be answered there. My answer

is that the kindergarten does not relieve us of
our burdens. There are some good kinder-
gartens, not many though. My own child has
attended two years. So far he has learned a
couple of hymns, how to cut out stars and doll
figures and paste them in a book—how to draw
some very crooked straight lines—how to be-
devil me because I don't say my prayers and
don't go to church. He can read some because
his mother and I have taught him, he can
hammer and saw and do a million things with
his hands which he did not learn at kindergarten. He is organized along many lines
—canoes, automobiles, motor boats, and farm
life. We have tried honestly to answer
every question he has ever asked us. We go
further at times. We pump him in the sense
that we try to draw out questions and try to
get *him to formulate in words* the things that
have happened to him during the day. Pretty
soon we began to glean from him what the
outside is giving him—Grace says this—Annie
says that. This procedure gives us a chance

to supplement, correct and elaborate. Since we take all the misinformation we glean from him as a matter of course, since nothing is called "naughty" or "vulgar" or "unrefined" or "not nice" but everything judged on the basis of accuracy or completeness, we keep him opening up to us. The moment we show ourselves shocked or angered or begin to berate the older playmates, that moment we are lost. Our child no longer uses us as a clearing house.

It is very easy, *if you start early,* to form a "talk it out club" with your children. When this club is going well it is a safeguard to health and sanity. The chance that *anything can go "wrong" with a child* so brought up is enormously minimized. The only danger there is, is the danger of too strong fixation by the child upon the father or mother but this can be handled as I pointed out on page 82 ff.

The types of questions children ask differ markedly—age, environment, whether older children are about, whether a new baby is soon to appear or has just appeared—all are factors. Here is a kind of running account of the actual questions asked by a youngster during the 2–5 year period. His mother gives the report.

"At two years of age Richard was in the habit of coming into my room every morning and staying for awhile. He usually played while I took my bath and came in and out of the bathroom—sometimes he would play at helping me take my bath. From the time he was twenty months of age he knew the names of various parts of the body—such as, stomach, arms, legs, hands, breasts, penis. Even after he had had breasts explained to him he often remarked on them just by pointing his finger at them or touching them and saying: 'What's that, breasts?' Throughout this period his interest kept alive in them. Not in all probability for hidden Freudian reasons but because of the fact that they were so different from any organ of his own. He wanted to know at the age of two what the navel was called. After it was explained to him he still asked questions for several weeks: 'What's that—navy?' to which I always answered 'Yes, navel.' Occasionally he would point to the pubic hairs and say 'What's that—hair?' Then he often touched the hair on my head and repeated 'Hair too.' These questions were no more frequent than millions of others he asked about his toys, shoes, clothes or other objects in daily use.

"At about this time I was six months pregnant and Richard remarked on the size of my stomach. I told him that there was a little baby in there. When the baby moved I used to call Richard in and let him feel it but he never thought to ask to feel it. His interest in the baby was very fleeting. One day he asked how it was going to get out. I explained in some detail—whereupon he said, 'Oh,' and that was all.

"Before the second child was born and for some time afterwards I was studying over a book on obstetrics. I occasionally showed

Richard pictures of the babies inside the mother. He seemed to understand it very well and one day I came in while he was showing a little friend a picture as he said of a 'baby borning out of his mama' (3 years of age then).

"After my second baby was born Richard saw him nursing immediately upon my return from the hospital. He noticed it and laughed. He never watched the process very closely. After about the third time he saw it, he just took it for granted. There was never the slightest sign of jealousy or resentment. Several times the following year he asked me if *he had a baby in his stomach.* Each time I told him the same thing—'only women have children.' Then one day he asked 'why' so I told him that their bodies were different from men's bodies—that women had a tiny egg in their bodies. That from this egg (when fertilized by the father) the tiny body of a baby began to develop—showing him in the book on obstetrics the changes in its form. Then he

asked how the baby ate and I told him, showing him his navel and telling him it was once
part of a tiny tube which connected him with
his mother and that through it he got liquid
food from the mother. He didn't get all of the
explanation but enough to satisfy his questions
for the time being.

"One day when the second baby was about
four months old, Richard asked me why I went
to the hospital to have Bobby. I told him how
difficult it was to bear a child and that sometimes a doctor had to help the baby out. And
then he asked how I knew when to go—which
I explained to him in detail. For some time
thereafter his questions stopped (possibly due
to instructions from an older child in the
neighborhood). Once in a while he referred
to the hospital and babies in the stomach.

"Shortly after his 3rd birthday he came
in while his father was undressed. He has
asked numerous times when he would get hair
on his body and when his own male organs
would grow up. We always told him that hair

would grow in time, pointing to the tiny hairs already present on his body.

"The only other interest during this year was in the body of his nurse. He asked if he could see her legs and also the legs of the cook. I had previously asked them to answer all of his questions naturally. He also wanted to see his nurse take a bath. We told him that if he was up some time when she took a bath he could see her but that there was no reason why she should take a bath especially for his benefit. He repeatedly asked if he could marry her and begged many times to be allowed to sleep with her. One night we allowed him to sleep in the same room with her. He was quite pleased but never asked to do it again. During the early part of his 5th year his chief interest was in himself. 'When will I be able to shave and when will I get more hair on my body?' Every summer we put the children out in the sun naked—in the back yard. Very often he wanted to run around the house naked. One day, when slightly over 4 years of age, he asked why he ever had to wear clothes. I told him it was all right for him to go without them at home but that lots of other people didn't live that way and that when he was out he would have to live the way other people lived. This seemed to strike him as being reasonable. When bathing at home he always invited any guests in when he took a bath.

"One day when Richard was 4½ a friend of mine visited me who was soon to have a baby. We told Richard about it. He clapped his hands and said 'Goody, goody—bring *her* out to play with me.' Within the past week the baby arrived. When I told him about it he said, 'When did it come?'

" 'About twelve o'clock last night.'

" 'Oh, did she have to wake up in the middle of the night?' So again I patiently explained that she was awake because one had pains a long time before. 'Why did she have a baby?'

" 'Because she wanted one.'

" 'How did she get it?'

" 'It grew from the egg inside of her.'

"About a month ago (4 years 10 months) he went up to see a little baby about three months old and the mother said to him, 'Look what a lovely little brother the stork brought Amy.' When he came home he said, 'Mrs. L—— said the stork brought Amy's brother.' I said, 'Well you know better than that, don't you?' He laughed and said, 'Well she said so.' So I said, 'Well now you tell me the truth,' and he said, 'Did it come in her stomach?' with some uncertainty of conviction. So again I told him that it did and asked him if he didn't remember how large my stomach was when Bobby was born. He said 'Yes' but I think it was vague.

"About a month after this he *'blocked'* all questions about babies. This was something new. I said to him, 'Richard, what do you know about where babies come from?'

" 'I don't know anything.'

" 'But don't you want to talk about it any more?'

" 'No.'

" 'Why not?'

" 'Anna says it isn't nice to talk about babies.'

"A few diagrams on paper brought him over to my chair. Then a little talk about how birds lay their eggs in nests, then sit on them to keep them warm—then about how the whole brood hatches out after three weeks, broke down the last resistance. This brought questions about lions and tigers. Finally he took paper and pencil and began to draw lions and tigers with eggs inside them developing into baby lions and tigers."

Rarely does the child under 7 connect the father with the having of children unless he is prompted from the outside. There is no reason if the question is asked even before this why you should not tell him the story of how the egg in the mother becomes fertilized. It is a story easily and simply told and it is a thousand times better for you to tell it than to have the hoodlum around the corner beat you to it. When children are brought up around white rats and rabbits it is very easy to explain the rôle the male plays. The sex act in these animals should be specifically pointed out to the children and explained. Ensuing pregnancy and the delivery of young should be watched by the children.

Fortunately the child at about this age begins to read. It becomes increasingly possible to give him considerable organization in this way. At 10 the boy or girl can begin upon a simple physiology or biology—but always read with him and discuss everything with him after the reading. Reading and discussion should begin not later than 11 years of age on the whole subject of *reproduction*—the *changes* that come to the boy and the girl at puberty and above all on the problem of *venereal disease*. They need a competent physician's hands here. But choose your physician. He should give them facts. Facts are hard enough to face without having the physician scare them.

It seems to me that we should develop sex

knowledge in our children as rapidly as they can take it in. The old theory was to wait until the child's own questions came naturally. I don't believe in this. The medical profession has practically ruled diphtheria out by innoculating the child against it. The germ cannot get a foothold in the immunized child. So it is with children who have full information. Street corner talk loses its punch.

The child whose knowledge has been made full and complete passes into adolescence, the years from 12–18, without shock. When the child is inadequately prepared these years are years of Stygian darkness and fear. Adolescence should not be any different from any other stretch of years. This period is apparently harder for the boy than the girl. For some reason, possibly due to anatomical factors, masturbation is more prevalent during this period among boys than among girls. A mother who lets her daughters come to puberty, or a father his sons, without telling them the facts about this subject are cruel in the extreme.

Masturbation is not, however, a problem that begins in puberty. For the parent it is a problem which begins at birth. Children as young as 6 months begin it. If wisely handled it produces little disturbance in children before puberty. As the children get older and more highly organized the trouble begins. Parents tell them that it is awful—unclean—that it will destroy manhood and womanhood, that it will produce insanity. Then conflict begins. The habit is rarely broken at puberty and the adolescent goes through purgatory. He wonders if people suspect—he begins to watch himself for signs of lack of sanity—restlessness, insomnia, anxiety beset him. The girl or boy with prudish parents has to go through this Gethsemane alone.

How does the wise parent handle it? Almost from birth watchfulness begins. Hygienic care is insisted upon—irritations are kept down. The tightness of the foreskin must be watched —your physician should be consulted about it (circumcision may be indicated). Clothing should not be tight or too warm. Covers should not be too heavy or too numerous. Their hands should be watched. It is easy to get young children to form the habit of sleeping with their hands outside the covers—this is especially important. Persistent tree climbing, the popular sport of sliding down the banister—and the earlier dangling astride the father's leg—are all forms of activity that must be scrutinized somewhat. Their association with older children should be watched—and this, heaven knows, is the hardest problem of all. A child of 6 or 8 badly brought up associating with your child of 4 can fast make a wreck of your most careful efforts.

Later comes verbal organization. "That is not for handling—it is to be used now for just one purpose"—telling him what that purpose is. Here you are likely to be met with a stubborn argument. "Why can't I play with it— it is mine" (this an actual statement from a two year old). It can always be met with the statement that father or mother does not do this. Another procedure is to give the child a toy to play with (substitutive activity). But when toys are given it should be seen to that the play activity started with them does not unduly prolong the act of sitting on the toilet.

In spite of it all, this form of sex outlet will be utilized during adolescence. If you have followed your child's organization—been a part of it from infancy, you can talk freely about this with him. Scaring the adolescent about it is little short of criminal. This was the old method indulged in by parents and physicians. Imagine my astonishment one day in talking with a state psychiatrist about this problem. "I believe," he said, "in scaring them nearly to death. When I was 15 my father nearly scared me to death about this and it was effective. Tell 'em it will make 'em crazy." Fortunately there are few psychiatrists today who are so benighted. Nearly all of the enlightened physicians admit that not too frequent masturbation produces no physiological disturbance and no general behavior difficulties if there has been no poor instruction. Straight-forward talks every now and then with your son or daughter in which you point out that this act is *not necessary*—that it is a kiddish trick—the sooner broken the better if he or she is ever to be like other grown up men and women is your best procedure. If it produces little physiological harm, why bother about it?

There is one cogent reason against it and this can be pointed out to the intelligent adolescent in this way— "Don't you see that you are doing this so persistently that it takes up your time and energy *for doing and learning the other things* which will help you get along in life?—That it takes up your thoughts (and these for the behaviorist are acts) and gives you no time for organizing your life?—That it makes you unfriendly—makes you withdraw from other people's society? You can't expect to have friends if you have no time or thought for them."

The most important reason of all for breaking this habit is this: *If it is persisted in too long and practiced too often it may make heterosexual adjustment difficult or impossible. This is as true for young women as for young men.* This fact can be communicated but should not be used to frighten the adolesent.

Another set of situations has to be watched very closely. Girls should not have as companions only girls. Boys should not have as companions only boys. The majority of parents somehow feel safe if their boys run with boys and their girls run with girls. Nothing is further from the truth and the parents who resign their girls only to girl companions, girl scouting organizations, the Y. W. C. A.; and their boys to boys' camps, Boy Scouts and to the Y. M. C. A.—without knowing how they are run and by whom—without frequent "talk it out contacts" with their children—are pursuing an unwise and dangerous course of conduct.

The boy brought up only or mainly with boys is very likely to want club life and to be with men all his days. He may marry, but home gives him very little stimulation. His wife and children see little of him. This forms a poor basis for marriage. And this is only the least alarming of the possible pictures. The boy so brought up may shy away completely from marriage and turn to men for a sex outlet. This is called *homosexuality*. Exactly the same is true with women. Our whole social fabric is woven so as to make all women slightly homosexual. Girls hold hands, kiss, embrace, sleep together, etc. Mothers think this is a natural kind of relationship.

We feel reasonably sure now that homosexuality is an affair of nurture rather than original nature. When our children deviate from standard sex conduct along these lines, we'd like to think that it is due to hereditary or to constitutional factors and hence not our fault.

Professor Moss, of George Washington University, made some recent experiments along these lines with animals. He placed a male rat brought up in a mixed colony with other males and females at one end of a box. At the other end he placed a female behind a wire fence. Before the male could get to the female he had to pass over an electrically charged network of wires on the floor. The strength of the current could be increased to the point where the male *just would not walk over it*. This gave a measure of the "punishment" he would take to get to the female. It was found that he would take considerable punishment to reach her.

Will the female take an equal amount of punishment to get at the male when the experiment is reversed? Moss's experiments show that they will take even greater punishment. (In the light of this little lesson in biology isn't it ridiculous for a mother to think that her girls are not interested in the males? It is a good sign when they are.)

The next experiment of Prof. Moss showed that if the males *are brought up only with other males they will not take any punishment to get at the female. In other words the female is no stimulus* to a male so brought up.

Certainly the results here, as well as those coming from the field of psychopathology, indicate that boys and girls should be brought up together so that enduring friendship and comradeship may spring up naturally.

The hardest problem of all in sex instruction is the preparation of one's children for love and marriage. (Unfortunately, since we have failed them, they are fast taking this out of our hands). Because the great majority of parents have never solved this problem for themselves they rarely help their children with it. No mother can tell her daughter all she ought to know about marriage the day before the marriage takes place. No father in one interview can tell his son how to be a successful and skillful sex companion for his wife—*nor even how to start to learn to be.*

And yet the happiness of the newly married is often wrecked within the first few weeks of marriage for lack of fundamentals.

Every college and university should have a department where sex instruction can be pursued by students during their 18th, 19th and 20th years. It should include instruction on the prevalence and dangers of venereal disease. Whether individuals who have once had a venereal disease should marry even if a "cure" has been effected (a very important question since, according to venereal disease statistics, about 70% of the male population either has or has had a venereal disease).

This department of a college should instruct both the young men and the young women in the *ars amandi;* for certainly love is an art and not an instinct. To achieve skill in this art requires time, patience, willingness to learn from each other, frankness in discussion and above all knowledge of what to expect.

Until the colleges can put this form of instruction in safer hands, we parents must continue to teach our children about love and marriage. But isn't it advisable for all of us to increase our own knowledge by first divesting ourselves of our own prudery and then studying the subject as we would any other scientific problem?

CHAPTER SEVEN

THE BEHAVIORIST'S APOLOGIA

A FTER this brief survey of the psychological care of infant and child the behaviorist hastens to admit that he has no "ideals" for bringing up children. He does not know how the ideal child should be brought up. The standards imposed by present society are not his standards. He is often criticised for not rushing in with plans for instructing children how to grow up in accordance with the specifications of his Utopia.

As a matter of fact there are as many ways of bringing up the child as there are civilizations. The behaviorist might advocate a very different manual of psychological care for the Chinese infant from the one he would prescribe for native Australian or African offspring. There is no ideal system of civilization—there are only actual civilizations, hence the child must be brought up along practical lines to fit a given civilization. Had the child we picture here grown up in the days of Cotton Mather, he would probably have spent most of his time in the stocks for insubordination. Had he been brought up at the time of the French Revolution, he would have been looked upon as a gentleman who did not understand the virtues of fire and rape, and if in the times of the Crusaders, as a worker fit only to be farrier or artisan. Finally, had he reached adulthood in the balmy military days of Huguenot versus Catholic, he would have been called by both parties a wicked heretic only fit to be burned at the stake.

We must face the fact that standards of training are changing as our civilization changes—and civilization is changing under our very eyes at a far more rapid rate than it has ever changed in the past. I do not except here the changes that went on at the time of the French Revolution or those that are going on in the Soviet Republic. In both these instances the changes affected mainly the nobility. I believe that the internal structure of our American civilization is changing from top to bottom more rapidly and more fundamentally than most of us dream of. Consequently today less than ever before, is it expedient to bring up a child in accordance with the fixed molds that our parents imposed upon us.

We have tried to sketch in the foregoing chapters a child as free as possible of sensitivities to people and one who, almost from birth, is relatively independent of the family situation. Naturally we have had to give the child customary manners and to build up conventions in him, and to give him a daily personal routine since he must have such habits if his guts (emotional equipment) are to give him time to do anything else.

Above all, we have tried to create a problem-solving child. We believe that a problem-solving technique (which can be trained) plus boundless absorption in activity (which can also be trained) are behavioristic factors which have worked in many civilizations of the past and which, so far as we can judge, will work equally well in most types of civilizations that are likely to confront us in the future.

INDEX

INDEX

A

Acquisition, of fear, 24
Acquisitiveness, 37
Activities, early morning, 122
Activity, absorption in, 187
  interference with, 34
Adolescence, 173
Aluminum mits, 139
Anger, 37, 42
Appropriation, 37
Avoidance reactions, 42, 56

B

Babies, normal, 35
Babinski, reflex, 20
Balance, reaction to loss of, 27
Bathe, learning to, 108
Bathing, 115
Bed-wetting, prevention of, 131

Behavior, lack of instinctive, 37
  rage, 88
Behaviorist's, apologia, 184
  belief about hereditary organization, 41
Birth, activities at, 35
  equipment at, 36, 37

C

Capacity, 41
Care, night and day, 113
Caressing, of children, 44
Characteristics, 41
Child, lack of knowledge of, 13
  reaction of to injury, 56
Cleanliness, 37
Climbing, 37
Coddling, 75, 80, 83, 86
Conditioned, fears, 29, 53
  rage responses, 94
Conditioning, of love response, 74

H

Habits, nest, 85
Hampering, 90
Handedness, acquired or
 inherited, 19
 test for, 19
Head, steadiness of, 21
Heredity, 15
Holding, 91
Homosexuality, 178
Hospital, lying-in, 17
Hunting, 37

I

Incontinence, 128
Infant, culture of, 16
Infants, hardy nature of,
 17
 laboratory study of, 17
Imitation, 37
Instinctive love, lack of at
 birth, 72
Instincts, James' list of,
 37
Interference with activity,
 cause of rage, 34
Interference with move-
 ment, 90
Invalidism, 76

J

Jealousy, 37

K

Kindergarten, 161
Kisses, parental, 70
Kissing, of infants, 14, 44
Kleptomania, 37

L

Laboratory work, preju-
 dice against, 16
Love, 37˙
 and marriage, instruc-
 tion in, 181
 no instinctive of mother,
 43
 of mother, 69, 80

M

Manipulation, 79
Marriage, 86
 instruction in, 181
Masturbation, 174
Mental, constitution, 41
Modesty, 37
Monkeys, behavior of
 young, 36
 lack of fear of, 25
Mothers, modern, 12
 over-devotion of, 11

N

Nature, of fear reaction,
 51

Family in America

AN ARNO PRESS / NEW YORK TIMES COLLECTION

Abbott, John S. C. **The Mother at Home:** Or, The Principles of Maternal Duty. 1834.

Abrams, Ray H., editor. **The American Family in World War II.** 1943.

Addams, Jane. **A New Conscience and an Ancient Evil.** 1912.

The Aged and the Depression: Two Reports, 1931–1937. 1972.

Alcott, William A. **The Young Husband.** 1839.

Alcott, William A. **The Young Wife.** 1837.

American Sociological Society. **The Family.** 1909.

Anderson, John E. **The Young Child in the Home.** 1936.

Baldwin, Bird T., Eva Abigail Fillmore and Lora Hadley. **Farm Children.** 1930.

Beebe, Gilbert Wheeler. **Contraception and Fertility in the Southern Appalachians.** 1942.

Birth Control and Morality in Nineteenth Century America: Two Discussions, 1859–1878. 1972.

Brandt, Lilian. **Five Hundred and Seventy-Four Deserters and Their Families.** 1905. Baldwin, William H. **Family Desertion and Non-Support Laws.** 1904.

Breckinridge, Sophonisba P. **The Family and the State:** Select Documents. 1934.

Calverton, V. F. **The Bankruptcy of Marriage.** 1928.

Carlier, Auguste. **Marriage in the United States.** 1867.

Child, [Lydia]. **The Mother's Book.** 1831.

Child Care in Rural America: Collected Pamphlets, 1917–1921. 1972.

Child Rearing Literature of Twentieth Century America, 1914–1963. 1972.

The Colonial American Family: Collected Essays, 1788–1803. 1972.

Commander, Lydia Kingsmill. **The American Idea.** 1907.

Davis, Katharine Bement. **Factors in the Sex Life of Twenty-Two Hundred Women.** 1929.

Dennis, Wayne. **The Hopi Child.** 1940.

Epstein, Abraham. **Facing Old Age.** 1922. New Introduction by Wilbur J. Cohen.

The Family and Social Service in the 1920s: Two Documents, 1921–1928. 1972.

Hagood, Margaret Jarman. **Mothers of the South.** 1939.

Hall, G. Stanley. **Senescence:** The Last Half of Life. 1922.

Hall, G. Stanley. **Youth:** Its Education, Regimen, and Hygiene. 1904.

Hathway, Marion. **The Migratory Worker and Family Life.** 1934.

Homan, Walter Joseph. **Children & Quakerism.** 1939.

Key, Ellen. **The Century of the Child.** 1909.

Kirchwey, Freda. **Our Changing Morality:** A Symposium. 1930.

Kopp, Marie E. **Birth Control in Practice.** 1934.

Lawton, George. **New Goals for Old Age.** 1943.

Lichtenberger, J. P. **Divorce:** A Social Interpretation. 1931.

Lindsey, Ben B. and Wainwright Evans. **The Companionate Marriage.** 1927. New Introduction by Charles Larsen.

Lou, Herbert H. **Juvenile Courts in the United States.** 1927.

Monroe, Day. **Chicago Families.** 1932.

Mowrer, Ernest R. **Family Disorganization.** 1927.

Reed, Ruth. **The Illegitimate Family in New York City.** 1934.

Robinson, Caroline Hadley. **Seventy Birth Control Clinics.** 1930.

Watson, John B. **Psychological Care of Infant and Child.** 1928.

White House Conference on Child Health and Protection. **The Home and the Child.** 1931.

White House Conference on Child Health and Protection. **The Adolescent in the Family.** 1934.

Young, Donald, editor. **The Modern American Family.** 1932.